Acupoint Location Guide
Revised Edition

By Alon Lotan B.Sc.T.E.

Preface by Prof. Ralph L. Carasso
NCCAOM Approved Abbreviations

- etsem -

For my son Aviv Ranen,
whom I hope will grow up to be
a happy, peaceful and fulfilled person.

ISBN 965-222-735-8
DANA Code: 800-800008

Copyright © 1995 by Alon Lotan
All rights reserved
Published by Etsem - Alon Lotan
info@etsem.co.il
Yodfat, D.N. Misgav, 20180, Israel
Tel: 972 4 9800395
Order through www.etsem.co.il

First Printing - 2000

I Would Like to Thank

My father, Amram Lotan
who was of great support and aid in every step of this book's publication.

Tzvika Na'amani, Dipl.Ac.
a wonderful "hevruta", whose help is tangible in every page.

Ofer Raz N.D., C.A.
who was a demanding teacher and encouraged excellence.

Prof. Ralph L. Carasso
who reviewed the book and gave me his blessing.

Dr. Charlie Xue
David Twicken Ph.D., L.Ac.
Debra Duncan
Elizabeth Kwee Ja Ohm, O.M.D., L.Ac.
Haihe Tian Ph.D., M.D.
Harvey Kaltsas, D.O.M., D.Ac., A.P., Dipl. Ac.
Dr. Jack Richman
Kevin V. Ergil M.A., M.S., L.Ac., Dipl.Ac.
Malvin Finkelstein
Reuven Barak, M.D.
Ronald Sokolsky Dipl.Ac.
Shen Ping Liang Ph.D., L.Ac.
Stuart Watts L.Ac., O.M.D., N.D.
Dr. Winifred A. Adams
who contributed their time, constructive criticism, and help in advancing the book.

Ariel Ring
Steven Stevenson
who made the book reader-friendly.

Kazuo Ishii
for the calligraphy on the book cover.

Warning

**Do not insert needles or otherwise manipulate the acupoints
unless you are trained.**
Incorrect acupuncture can result in complications ranging from bleeding, injuring a
nerve, artery or muscle, to grand mal epileptic seizures. Familiarity with acupoints is
only one aspect. Good results in acupuncture requires advanced studies which are not
within the scope of this Guide!

Preface

This book answers one of the most critical problems in acupuncture: how to accurately locate the acupoints.

It is imperative to practice exact point location. Inaccurate needling may not only cause ineffective treatment, but may even lead to harm (e.g. penetration of blood vessels, injury to nerves, etc.). In addition, the location is closely related to one's body frame and structure - the points on the body of a slender woman are not the same as those of a heavy man, and both are different from those of a small child.

In this guide, Alon has found the perfect method of simplifying points location technique through the combination of unique, all new original illustrations and easy-to-follow text for each and every point on all the meridians.

Special attention was given to combine in every illustration all anatomical information (skin, muscle, artery and bone- if relevant, in best body posture) to guide the reader how to locate the point. The comparative maps and the Introduction section complement the text and the illustrations.

The creative combination of one who has practiced both acupuncture and shiatsu, along with a paramedic's anatomical know-how, and the talent of a designer, have culminated in this attractive, well-written and user-friendly book which can be used as a first-class guide for students as well as practitioners.

Prof. Ralph L. Carasso M.D., M.Sc.
Head, Complementary Medicine Outpatient Clinic
Head, Department of Neurology and Pain Clinic
Hillel Yaffe Medical Center, Hadera, Israel

Table of Contents

Meridians and Acupoints

The human body and its condition is the consequence of many interdependent processes: physical, chemical, genetic, mental, spiritual, energetic and others. The energetic process deals with the changes in the movement, strength, and location of Qi, which can be described as something between material and spiritual.

The Qi flows in many ways and on many levels; on each level it moves in a specific course as if flowing through a canal. The most external course, in which the Qi is most superficial, is on the muscle and tendon stratum. This course circulates the body three times before completing one cycle and beginning another. Furthermore, this cycle is divided into twelve sections, each called a meridian and each related to a specific organ. These twelve meridians are commonly divided into 4 groups of three: The three leg Yin meridians, starting at the toes and rising to the chest; three arm Yin meridians starting on the chest and ending at the fingers; three arm Yang meridians, starting at the fingers and running to the back; and three leg Yang meridians, ending at the toes. **This cyclic concept is illustrated in the diagram below**.

In order to understand the functions of each meridian, one must consider several factors, such as: the organ it relates to and the organ's physiological role in the body processes; the parts of the body through which it passes; the succeeding meridian (e.g. Heart succeeds Spleen) and the preceding one; its proximity to the front or back midlines, as well as to the upper or lower part of the body.

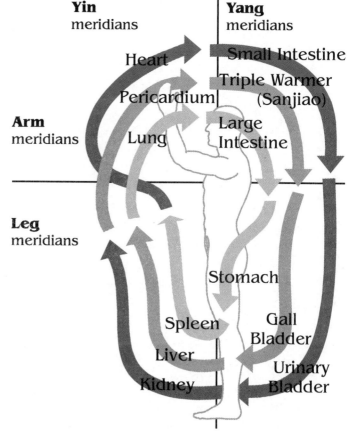

This basic scheme grows rich and complex. Each meridian branches, crossing organs, other meridians, and creating points of interaction. In addition, located on the meridians are indentations or openings. These concavities, which are generally more sensitive and through which Qi can be manipulated externally, are used as acupoints.

In order to understand the functions of an acupoint, one should consider factors such as: the meridian on which it is located and if other meridian branches cross it; the part of the body it is on and the other points located nearby; its proximity to the center of the body or to the tips of the extremities; as well as the point's special "intelligence" and features.

In addition to the twelve meridians mentioned above, there is another group which is commonly used in acu-medicine: the "Eight Extra Meridians". These eight are considered to be remnants of embryonic development.

Two of these are similar to the first group of twelve in that they have their own points that can be accessed and manipulated externally, but they differ in that they do not succeed or precede each other. Both rise up from the perineum and close their cycle by passing through each other. The Ren Mai (Conception Vessel) is located on the front midline and the Du Mai (Governing Vessel) is located on the back midline.

The remaining six meridians of the second group do not have their own points, but can be manipulated via specific points that are located on the first twelve. Although symmetrical in form like the first twelve meridians, these six have a different significance on right and left sides, and these differences are reversed in man and woman.

The access of meridians and the location of points is only one branch of the knowledge developed by traditional Chinese philosophers / doctors. The other two main branches are Chinese philosophy, based on Yin and Yang, and Chinese organ physiology. The braiding together of these three streams is an important step in understanding the action of acupoints, and will help manipulate them beneficially.

Meridian Biological Clock

Another aspect of the cyclical nature of the superficial meridians is the daily rotation in which each meridian has a time of maximum and minimum influence; e.g., the Spleen meridian is most influential between 9-11 AM, and least so between 9-11 PM.

The following diagram illustrates each meridian's dominant hours. The external circle represents daytime and the internal circle, nighttime. The meridians are represented by their abbreviations which are listed on p. 14.

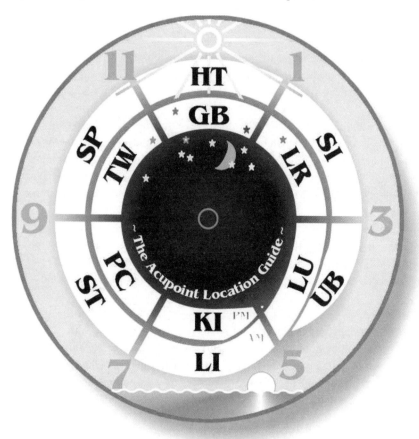

You can make your own meridian biological clock using a 200% photocopy* of this page and a simple clock mechanism.
Glue the photocopy onto a wooden board, cut along the perimeter, and make a hole in the center. Add the clock mechanism - and there you are!

---

* Please don't see permission to copy this page for this particular purpose as an invitation to ignore copyright laws.

The Guide Concept & Method

This Guide is a response to the need for clear, accessible descriptions of acupoint locations, a small but critical part of Chinese traditional knowledge. While a skilled acupuncturist can find the points through the sensitivity of the fingertips, anatomical descriptions can be an important aid to the student of acu-medicine.

This Revised Edition endeavors to provide easy to use directions for the exact locating of acupoints. Short, uniformly formatted textual descriptions are given alongside corresponding anatomical maps. The text and illustrations conform to the guidelines listed below.

Efforts have been made to include alternative locations of points which are mentioned in various sources. It does not presume to be a new approach, nor is it limited to one particular perspective.

This is the book I was looking for as a student. I hope you enjoy it.

Illustration Guidelines:

☆ The illustrations present all important anatomical details required for accurate location of the points.

☆ The different strata of the body: bones, muscles and tendons, skin, and arteries, are clearly delineated.

☆ The illustrations show the correct body posture for locating the points.

☆ All points are shown on the left side of the body, although they are found on both sides. Some illustrations show the point, untitled, also on the right side with additional anatomical aspects of the location.

☆ It is a good idea to use different colors to mark the various body structures in the illustrations, and to underline the corresponding text in the same color.

Text Guidelines:

☆ The names of the acupoints are given in Pinyin and in the NCCA abbreviations.

☆ The "Location" describes the point's horizontal and vertical position on the body, following the recommended body posture, if such is relevant.

☆ "Tips & References" provide the reader with additional information such as definitions from traditional sources, anatomically related structures and finger-tip search instructions.

☆ Most sources agree on the locations of points. "Alternative Locations" gives a variant location when such exists. Sources for alternative locations are given in the appendix, on p. 179.

☆ The text aims at accessibility to the general reader. All special terms ("cun" units, anatomical directions) are defined and illustrated in the Introduction. Names of anatomical structures are shown in the accompanying illustration.

☆ In order to keep the location definitions short and clear, simple terms have been substituted for the classical terminology. For example, a point located on the upper border of an organ is described as "superior to..." instead of "on the superior border of...". A point located directly above a site is described as "vertically superior to...", or, if a cun measure is given: "X cun superior to...".

Terminology of Anatomical Directions

The descriptions of point locations use the following anatomical terminology.

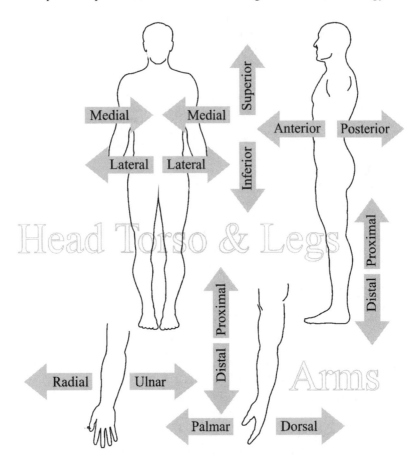

The Cun Unit of Measure

"Cun" is a unit of body measure, used in traditional Chinese sources, to help locate acupoints. The most important thing to remember about cun is that they are relative units, particular to the part of the body they divide. For example, there are 9 equal units on the nape of the neck between the ends of the two mastoid bones; each unit is one cun, and therefore each cun is 1/9 of the distance. This unit of cun is applicable only when looking for a point on the back of the neck of a particular person. It would be a mistake to try to locate a point on another part of the body, or on someone else's neck, with the same cun unit.

A list and illustrations of the body cun divisions appear on the following three pages.

Map of Body Cun Divisions

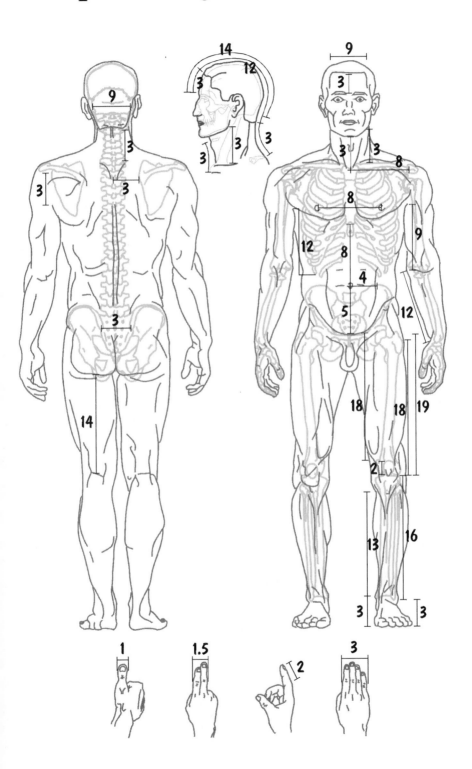

Table of Body Cun Divisions

A map of body cun divisions appears on the previous page (p. 11).

~ Head & Neck Cun Division ~

Body Part	Cun	Between...
Top midline	12	The forehead hairline and the neck hairline.
Top midline	14	The glabella, or eyebrow, and the occipit protuberance inferior border.
Forehead width	9	The two forehead hairline corners.
Forehead height	3	The glabella (eyebrow) and the forehead hairline.
Throat height	3	The clavicle medial end and the mandible angle, or between the hyoid and the manubrium superior border (when the head is straight).
Neck width	9	The inferior ends of the two mastoid bones.
Neck height	3	The neck hairline and the seventh cervical (C7) spinous process.

~ Torso Cun Division ~

Body Part	Cun	Between...
Front width	8	The two nipples.
Chest width	8	The front midline and the armpit (axillary) anterior end (when the arms lie straight alongside the body).
Chest width	8	The front midline and the acrominal tip.
Chest height	12	The armpit (axillary) and the 12th rib free end.
Abdomen width	4	The front midline and the rectus abdominis muscle's lateral border.
Upper abdomen height	8	The umbilicus center and the xiphisternal joint.
Lower abdomen height	5	The umbilicus center and the pubic symphysis superior border.
Back width	3	The back midline and the scapular spine medial end (when the arms lie straight alongside the body).
Lower back width	3	The two PSIS (posterior superior iliac spines).

~ Arm Cun Division ~

Body Part	Cun	Between...
Upper arm length	9	The front midline and the armpit (axillary) anterior end and the elbow (cubital) fold.
Lower arm length	12	The elbow (cubital) fold and the wrist (carpal) crease.
Back shoulder length	3	The acromion and the armpit (axillary) posterior end (when the arms lie straight alongside the body).

~ Leg Cun Division ~

Body Part	Cun	Between...
Thigh lateral length	19	The femur greater trochanter superior border and the knee (popliteal) fold and joint.
Thigh lateral length	18	The femur greater trochanter peak and the knee (popliteal) fold and joint.
Thigh medial length	18	The pubic symphysis superior border and the femur medial epicondyle superior border.
Knee length	2	The patella superior and inferior borders.
Lower leg lateral length	16	The lateral malleolus tip and the knee (popliteal) fold and joint.
Lower leg medial length	13	The medial malleolus tip and the tibial medial condyle inferior border.
Foot lateral height	3	The lateral malleolus tip and the sole.
Foot medial height	3	The medial malleolus tip and the sole.

~ Use of Fingers to Measure Cun ~

Cun	Between...
3	The two sides of the 4 fingers *, when they are joined together.
2	The pointing finger tip and the proximal interphalangeal joint (and fold).
1.5	The two sides* of the pointing and middle fingers, when they are joined together.
1	The two sides* of the thumb.

* Level with the proximal interphalangeal joints.

Meridian Abbreviations

Abbreviations are used to represent the twelve meridians, the front and back midline meridians, as well as their acupoints. In the table below the NCCA abbreviations, which are used in the Guide are listed first, followed by other common abbreviations.

Hand Taiyin	Lung	Lu / LU / L	Hand Yangming	Lge. Intestine	LI / Li
Foot Taiyin	Spleen	Sp / SP	Foot Yangming	Stomach	St / ST / S
Hand Shaoyin	Heart	H / HT / HE	Hand Taiyang	Sml. Intestine	SI / Si
Foot Shaoyin	Kidney	K / KI / KID	Foot Taiyang	Urinary Bladder	UB / BL / B
Hand Jueyin	Pericard	P / PC	Hand Shaoyang	Triple Warmer/	TW / SJ / T /
				Sanjiao	TH / TB
Foot Jueyin	Liver	Liv / LR / LV	Foot Shaoyang	Gall Bladder	GB / G
Ren Mai	Conception Vessel	CV / Ren / RN / REN	Du Mai	Governing Vessel	GV / Du / DU

Meridian Courses in the Body

The illustrations below show the courses of the fourteen meridians in the body.

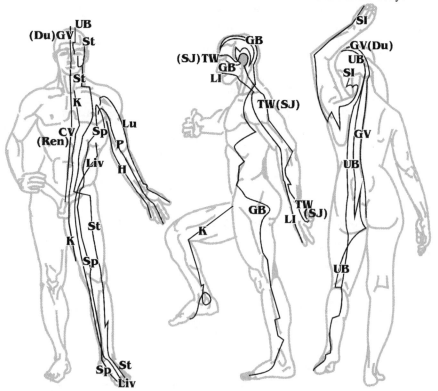

Scheme of Meridian Courses

The illustration below presents the 14 meridians and their basic cyclic relationship to one another. The cyclic relationship is made clear in the posture shown in the drawing, with the arms extended upward.

In this scheme, one can follow the idea of 6 stages which is used for understanding the activity of some points and the progression of some disorders. Note that the first stage is on the Yang side, running close to the back midline and GV(Du), and the sixth and deepest stage is on the Yin side, proximate to the front midline and CV(Ren).

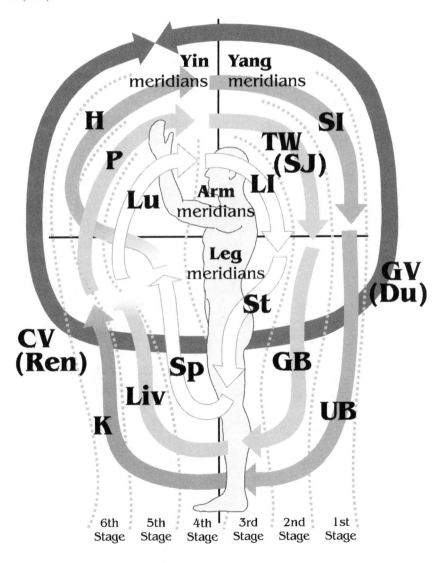

Lung Meridian

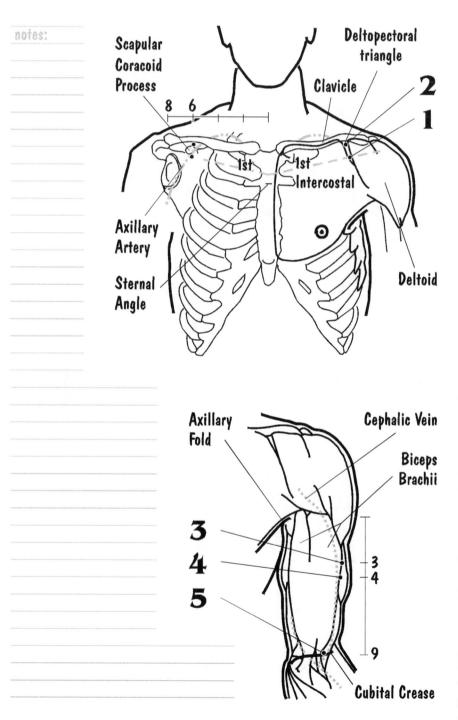

~ Acupoint Location Guide ~

Description:

~ Zhongfu ~ Lu 1

Location: 6 cun lateral to the front midline, on the line continuing laterally (and superior) from the 1st intercostal.

Tips & References: About 1 cun inferior (and lateral) to Lu 2.

☆　Medial to the deltoid muscle.

☆　The first intercostal is superior to the second rib which is level with the sternal angle.

☆　Medial to the axillary artery (search for the sensation of pulse).

☆　Search for the first deep depression that can be felt when moving inferiorly (and laterally) from Lu 2 along the deltoid border.

Basic Feature: Lu front 'Mu' collecting pt.. Interaction with Sp.

Note: ....

~ Yunmen ~ Lu 2

Location: Inferior to the clavicle, 6 cun lateral to the front midline.

Tips & References: Medial to the deltoid.

☆　In the superior part of the deltopectoral triangle depression.

☆　Superior to the scapular coracoid process (that can be felt only when pressing deeply).

☆　Easier to identify the anatomical structure when lifting the arm forward (flexion) against resistance.

Note: ....

~ Tianfu ~ Lu 3

Location: 3 cun distal to the anterior armpit crease (axillary fold), radial to the biceps brachii.

Basic Feature: Window to the Sky.

Note: ....

~ Xiabai ~ Lu 4

Location: 4 cun distal to the anterior armpit crease (axillary fold), radial to the biceps brachii.

Tips & References: 1 cun distal to Lu 3, 5 cun proximal to the cubital crease.

Note: ....

~ Chize ~ Lu 5

Location: When the elbow is slightly flexed, in the elbow fold (cubital crease), radial to the biceps brachii tendon.

Tips & References: Search for a small tendon radial to a big one (both are part of the biceps brachii). The point is radial to both.

☆　Easier to identify the anatomical structure when flexing the arm against resistance.

Basic Feature: 'He' sea, water, sedation pt..

Note: ....

Lung Meridian

notes:

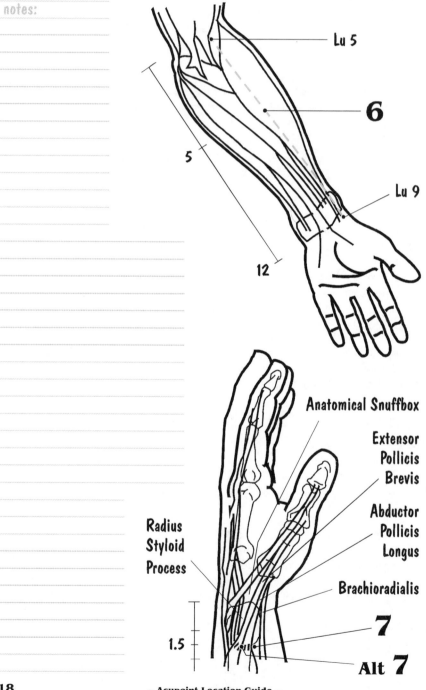

Lu 5

6

5

Lu 9

12

Anatomical Snuffbox

Extensor
Pollicis
Brevis

Abductor
Pollicis
Longus

Radius
Styloid
Process

Brachioradialis

7

1.5

Alt 7

Description:

~ Kongzui ~ Lu 6

Location: When the arm is straight and the palm faces the anterior (supination), on the line connecting Lu 9 with Lu 5, 5 cun distal to Lu 5.

Tips & References: Search for a split in the muscle that can be felt when moving proximally from Lu 9.

Basic Feature: 'Xi' accumulation pt..

Note: ....

~ Lieque ~ Lu 7

Location: Proximal to the radius styloid process, between the abductor pollicis longus and the brachioradialis.

Tips & References: Radial to the line that Lu 5, 6, 8, and 9 are on.

☆ 1.5 cun proximal to the carpal (wrist) crease.

☆ On the styloid process tip medial aspect.

☆ When crossing the hands so the webs between the thumbs and the index fingers are joined, the point is under the tip of the outside index finger. (This description may also indicate the alternative location given below).

Alternative Location: Proximal to the radius styloid process, between the abductor pollicis longus and the extensor pollicis brevis.

☆ 1.5 cun proximal to the cubital (wrist) fold.

☆ On the styloid process tip radial aspect.

☆ On the styloid process lateral aspect.

☆ When stretching the thumb upwards (extension) the two tendons at the wrist joint seem to be one and together they form the anatomical snuffbox medial border. This is a good place to search for the gap between them.

Basic Feature: 'Luo' connecting pt.. CV(Ren) opening pt.. Yinqiao (Yi-H) coupled pt.. Head and nape command pt..

Note: ....

Lung Meridian

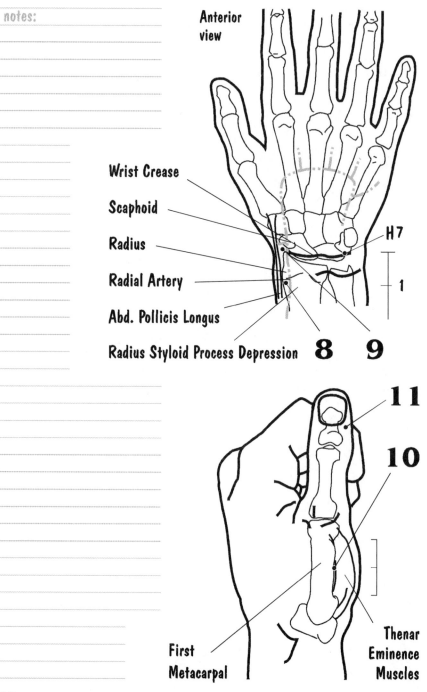

notes:

Anterior view

Wrist Crease

Scaphoid

Radius

Radial Artery

Abd. Pollicis Longus

Radius Styloid Process Depression

H7

1

8   **9**

11

10

First
Metacarpal

Thenar
Eminence
Muscles

Description:

~ Jingqu ~ Lu 8

Location: 1 cun proximal to the carpal (wrist) crease, radial to the radial artery.

Tips & References: Search for the sensation of pulse.

☆ On the line connecting Lu 9 with Lu 5.

☆ In the radius styloid process depression.

☆ Search for the first deep depression that can be felt when moving proximally from Lu 9.

Basic Feature: 'Jing' river, metal, horary pt..

Note: ....

~ Taiyuan ~ Lu 9

Location: In the carpal (wrist) joint, radial to the radial artery.

Tips & References: Search for the sensation of pulse.

☆ In the wrist transverse crease.

☆ Ulnar to the abductor pollicis longus.

☆ Between the radius and the scaphoid (carpal bone).

☆ Level with H 7*.

Basic Feature: 'Shu' stream, earth, tonification pt.. 'Yuan' source pt.. Blood vessels 'Hui' gathering pt..

Note: ....

~ Yuji ~ Lu 10

Location: On the radial aspect of the hand, midway on the first metacarpal bone neck (between the bone head border and the bone base border), palmar to the bone neck.

Tips & References: On the borderline between the palm skin and pigmented skin.

☆ Between the first metacarpal and the thenar eminence muscles.

☆ Palmar to a vertical slit on the first metacarpal bone.

Basic Feature: 'Ying' spring, fire pt..

Note: ....

~ Shaoshang ~ Lu 11

Location: 0.1 cun proximal to the thumb nail radial corner.

Tips & References: Proximal to the nail base.

Basic Feature: 'Jing' well, wood pt..

Note: ....

* See p. 64.

Large Intestine Meridian

notes:

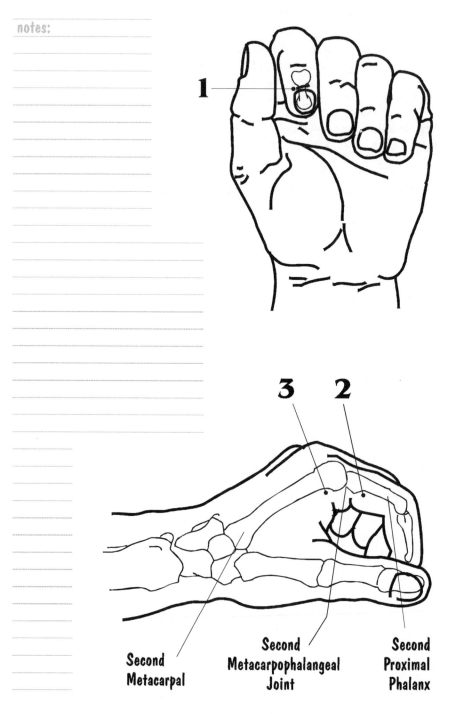

Second
Metacarpal

Second
Metacarpophalangeal
Joint

Second
Proximal
Phalanx

Description:

~ Shangyang ~ LI 1

Location: 0.1 cun proximal to the pointing (index) fingernail radial corner.
Tips & References: Proximal to the nail base.
Basic Feature: 'Jing' well, metal, horary pt..
Note: ....

~ Erjian ~ LI 2

Location: When the hand is in a loose fist (flexion), on the radial aspect of the index finger, distal to the 2nd proximal phalanx bone base, palmar to the bone neck.
Tips & References: On the borderline between the palm skin and pigmented skin.
☆　Distal to the 2nd metacarpophalangeal joint.
Basic Feature: 'Ying' spring, water, sedation pt..
Note: ....

~ Sanjian ~ LI 3

Location: When the hand is in a loose fist (flexion), proximal to the 2nd metacarpal bone head, palmar to the bone neck.
Tips & References: On the borderline between the palm skin and pigmented skin.
☆　Proximal to the 2nd metacarpophalangeal joint.
☆　In the gap between the bone and a muscle (first dorsal interosseous).
Basic Feature: 'Shu' stream, wood pt..
Note: ....

Large Intestine Meridian

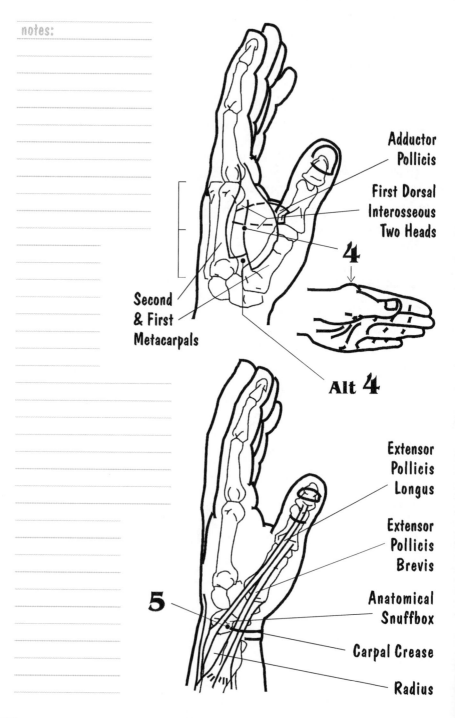

Adductor
Pollicis

First Dorsal
Interosseous
Two Heads

4

Second
& First
Metacarpals

Alt 4

Extensor
Pollicis
Longus

Extensor
Pollicis
Brevis

Anatomical
Snuffbox

Carpal Crease

Radius

5

Description:

~ Hegu ~ LI 4

Location: On the dorsal side of the hand, in the depression, between the two heads of the first dorsal interosseous muscle, level with the midpoint (between head and base) of the second metacarpal.

Tips & References: Ulnar to the midpoint between the center of the 1st and the center of the 2nd metacarpals.

☆ Proximal to the adductor pollicis.

☆ When the thumb and the pointing finger are joined, LI 4 is at the uppermost point, on the bulge that is formed.

☆ Search for the depression behind a stiff tissue that can be felt when moving proximally from the web margin.

☆ When placing the thumb of one hand on the web between the thumb and the index finger of the other hand, and the transverse crease of the thumb is on top of the web margin, LI 4 is under the thumb's tip. (This description may indicate the alternative location given below).

Alternative Location: On the dorsal side of the hand, in the depression, between the two heads of the first dorsal interosseous muscle, distal to the first and second metacarpal bone bases.

Basic Feature: 'Yuan' source pt.. Face and mouth command pt..

Note: ....

~ Yangxi ~ LI 5

Location: In the carpal (wrist) joint, between the extensor pollicis longus and the extensor pollicis brevis tendons.

Tips & References: On the line continuing radially (and dorsally) from wrist crease.

☆ Search for the deepest point in the anatomical snuffbox that is formed when stretching the thumb upwards.

Basic Feature: 'Jing' river, fire pt..

Note: ....

Large Intestine Meridian

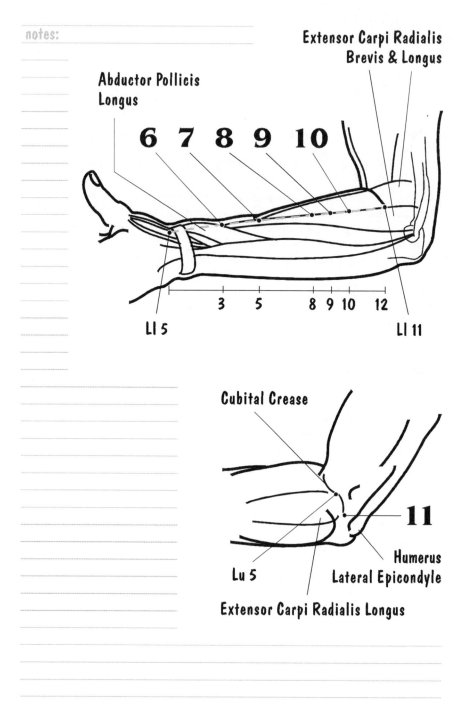

notes:

Abductor Pollicis Longus

Extensor Carpi Radialis Brevis & Longus

6 7 8 9 10

3   5   8 9 10 12

LI 5

LI 11

Cubital Crease

11

Lu 5

Humerus
Lateral Epicondyle

Extensor Carpi Radialis Longus

Description:

~ Pianli ~ LI 6

Location: When the hand rests on the belly, on the line connecting LI 5 with LI 11, 3 cun proximal to LI 5.

Tips & References: Search for the gap between the two tendons (abductor pollicis longus and extensor carpi radialis brevis).

Basic Feature: 'Luo' connecting pt..

Note: ....

~ Wenliu ~ LI 7

Location: When the hand rests on the belly, on the line connecting LI 5 with LI 11, 5 cun proximal to LI 5.

Tips & References: Easier to identify the body structure when the hand is fisted.

Basic Feature: 'Xi' accumulation pt..

Note: ....

~ Xialian ~ LI 8

Location: 8 cun proximal to LI 5, on the line connecting LI 5 with LI 11.

Tips & References: Easier to identify when the hand rests on the belly.

☆ Between the two tendons: extensor carpi radialis brevis and longus.

Note: ....

~ ShangLian ~ LI 9

Location: 9 cun proximal to LI 5, on the line connecting LI 5 with LI 11.

Tips & References: Easier to identify when the hand rests on the belly.

☆ 3 cun distal to the elbow fold (cubital crease).

☆ Between the two tendons: extensor carpi radialis brevis and longus.

☆ Search for the depression that can be felt when the hand rests on the belly, moving proximally along the radial-lateral aspect of the lower arm.

Note: ....

~ Shousanli ~ LI 10

Location: 10 cun proximal to LI 5, on the line connecting LI 5 with LI 11.

Tips & References: 2 cun distal to the elbow fold (cubital crease).

☆ Between the two tendons: extensor carpi radialis brevis and longus.

☆ Search for the depression that can be felt when the hand rests on the belly, moving gently, proximally along the radial-lateral aspect of the lower arm.

Basic Feature: St upper 'He' sea pt.. "Arm Three Miles."

Note: ....

~ Quchi ~ LI 11

Location: When the elbow is flexed, midway between Lu 5 and the humerus lateral epicondyle tip.

Tips & References: On the lateral end of the elbow (cubital) crease.

☆ Between the two tendons: extensor carpi radialis brevis and longus.

☆ Search for the gap between the soft and hard tissues.

Basic Feature: 'He' sea, earth, tonification pt..

Note: ....

Large Intestine Meridian

notes:

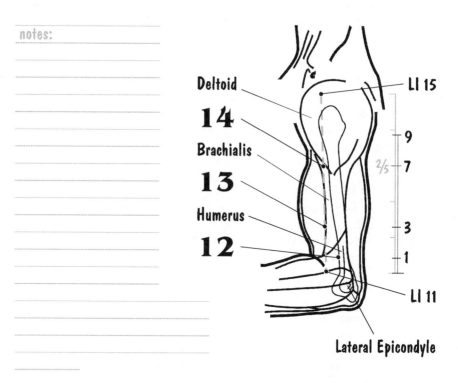

Deltoid

14

Brachialis

13

Humerus

12

LI 15

9

7 2/5

3

1

LI 11

Lateral Epicondyle

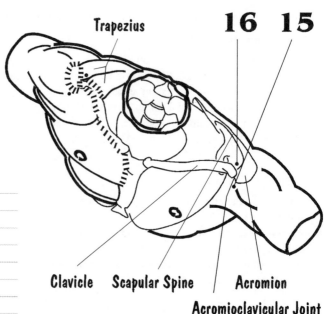

Trapezius

16 15

Clavicle   Scapular Spine   Acromion

Acromioclavicular Joint

Description:

~ Zhouliao ~ LI 12

Location: When the elbow is bent, on the lateral aspect of arm, anterior to the humerus, 1 cun superior (and lateral) to LI 11.

Tips & References: When the arm is straight, LI 12 is 2 cun proximal to LI 11.

☆   Search for a deep depression that can be felt when moving proximally from the lateral epicondyle toward the humerus anterior border.

Note: ....

~ Shouwuli ~ LI 13

Location: On the line connecting LI 11 with LI 15, 3 cun proximal to LI 11.

Tips & References: Anterior to hard tissue.

Note: ....

~ Binao ~ LI 14

Location: In the depression, anterior to the deltoid, about 0.5 cun superior (and anterior) to the (conspicuous) deltoid lower edge.

Tips & References: On the line connecting LI 11 with LI 15.

☆   In the gap, formed between the deltoid and the brachialis muscles.

☆   Easier to identify the anatomical structure when lifting the arm laterally (abduction) against resistance.

☆   About 7 cun proximal to LI 11.

☆   About 2/5 of the distance between LI 15 to LI 11.

☆   Anterior to the humerus.

Basic Feature: Many sources indicate interaction with SI, UB, and some indicate also interaction with Yangwei (Ya-L).

Note: ....

~ Jianyu ~ LI 15

Location: In the depression, about 0.3 cun inferior to the acromion anterior corner.

Tips & References: Search for the second small depression that can be felt when moving distally from the acromion corner

☆   When the arm is horizontal (abduction) and loose, two curved depressions appear on the shoulder. The point is in the anterior one, beneath the bone.

Basic Feature: Interaction with Yangqiao (Ya-H) and some sources indicate also interaction with SI and GB.

Note: ....

~ Jugu ~ LI 16

Location: In the depression, between the clavicle lateral end and the scapular spine.

Tips & References: Medial and posterior to the acromioclavicular joint.

☆   On the trapezius muscle.

☆   Search for the deep depression that can be felt when moving medially from the acromion toward the neck.

Basic Feature: Interaction with Yangqiao (Ya-H).

Note: ....

Large Intestin e Meridian

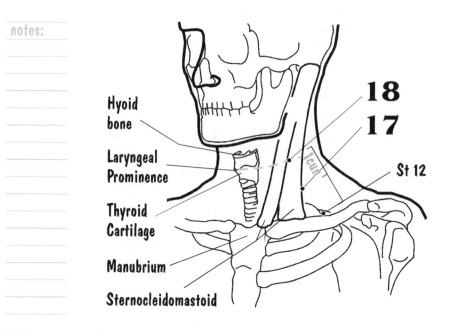

- Hyoid bone
- Laryngeal Prominence
- Thyroid Cartilage
- Manubrium
- Sternocleidomastoid

18
17
St 12

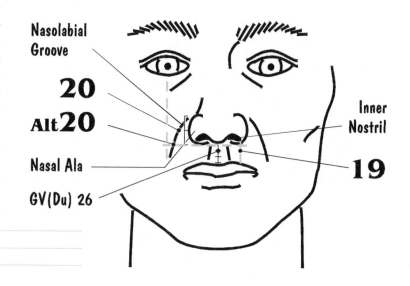

- Nasolabial Groove
- **20**
- **Alt 20**
- Nasal Ala
- GV(Du) 26

Inner Nostril

19

Description:

~ Tianding ~ LI 17

Location: Posterior to the sternocleidomastoid, level with 1 cun inferior to LI 18.

Tips & References: The sternocleidomastoid muscle of one side is more distinct when the head is turned to the other side and resisting a pressure applied (e.g. on the chin) from the first side.

☆ Midway between LI 18 to St 12*.

☆ One handbreadth posterior to the Adam's apple.

☆ The size of this cun*** is commonly bigger than other cuns measured on one's body.

Note: ....

~ Futu ~ LI 18

Location: Between the two heads of the sternocleidomastoid, level with the Adam's apple peak (laryngeal prominence).

Tips & References: The sternocleidomastoid muscle of one side is more distinct when the head is turned to the other side and resisting a pressure applied (e.g. on the chin) from the first side.

☆ On a line starting at the Adam's apple peak (laryngeal prominence) and parallel to the jaw.

☆ When the Adam's apple peak is difficult to identify, search for the peak location on the inferior border of the depression formed by the hyoid bone and the thyroid cartilage.

Basic Feature: Window to the Sky.

Note: ....

~ Kouheliao ~ LI 19

Location: Inferior to the inner nostril lateral border, level with 1/3 of the distance between the nostril root inferior border and the upper lip superior border.

Tips & References: The 1/3 distance should be measured on the front midline.

☆ Level with GV(Du) 26**.

☆ About 0.5 cun lateral to the front midline.

Note: ....

~ Yingxiang ~ LI 20

Location: In the nasolabial groove, level with the midpoint of the nasal ala lateral border.

Tips & References: The LI meridian is unique in that it crosses the midline and thus LI 20 is located on the opposite side.

Alternative Location: In the nasolabial groove, level with the nasal ala inferior border.

Basic Feature: Interaction with St.

Note: ....

* See p. 38.   ** See p. 172.
*** There are 3 cuns between the hyoid bone and the manubrium superior border, or otherwise, between the clavicle medial end and the mandible angle.

~ Points on Foot Yangming ~
Stomach Meridian

notes:

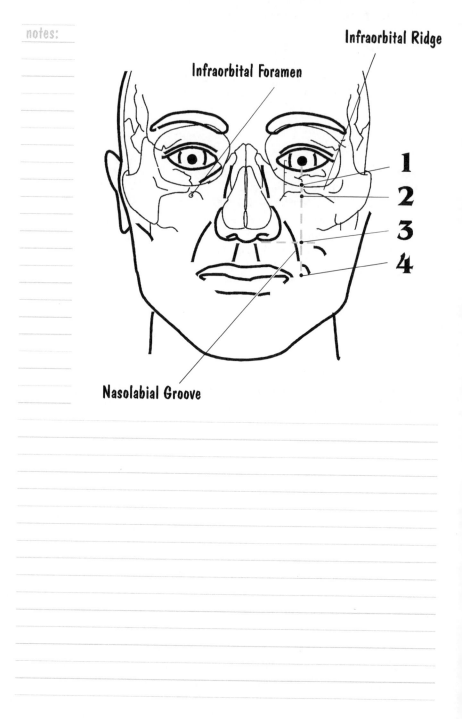

Infraorbital Ridge

Infraorbital Foramen

1
2
3
4

Nasolabial Groove

Description:

~ Chengqi ~ St 1

Location: When looking straight ahead, vertically inferior to the pupil center, superior to the infraorbital ridge.

Tips & References: Inferior to the eyeball.

☆ Search for a vertical slit on the infraorbital ridge.

Basic Feature: Interaction with CV(Ren) and Yangqiao (Ya-H).

Note: ....

~ Sibai ~ St 2

Location: On the infraorbital foramen.

Tips & References: Vertically inferior to St 1.

☆ When looking straight ahead, about 1 cun inferior to the pupil center.

☆ When looking straight ahead, the distance between St 1 and St 2 is half of the distance between the pupil and St 1.

☆ Search for a first small depression inferior to the center of the infraorbital ridge.

Note: ....

~ Juliao ~ St 3

Location: When looking straight ahead, vertically inferior to the pupil center, level with the nasal ala inferior border.

Tips & References: St 1, 2, 3 and 4 create a straight, vertical line.

☆ Lateral to the nasolabial groove.

Basic Feature: Interaction with Yangqiao (Ya-H).

Note: ....

~ Dicang ~ St 4

Location: When looking straight ahead, vertically inferior to the pupil center, level with the mouth corner.

Tips & References: About 0.4 cun lateral to the mouth corner.

☆ On the line continuing the nasolabial groove.

☆ When the lips are tight, at the tip of the bulge that is formed.

Basic Feature: Interaction point with LI, Yangqiao (Ya-H) and some sources indicate also interaction with CV(Ren).

Note: ....

~ Points on Foot Yangming ~

Stomach Meridian

notes:

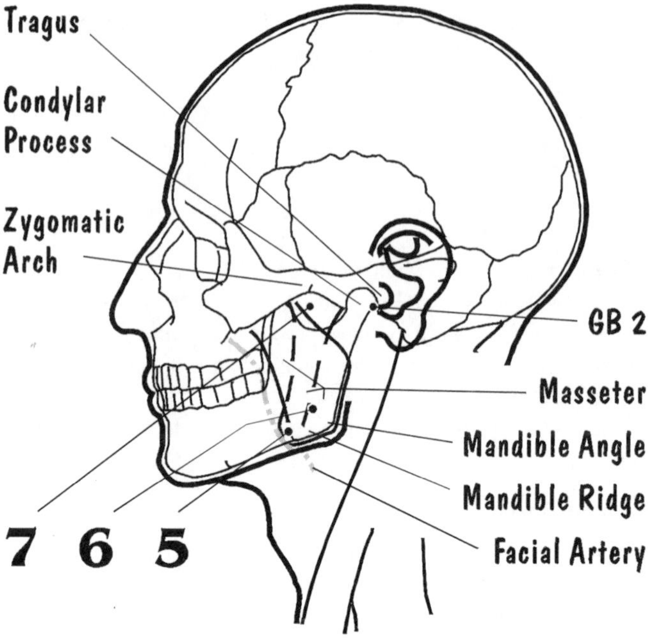

Tragus
Condylar Process
Zygomatic Arch
GB 2
Masseter
Mandible Angle
Mandible Ridge
Facial Artery
7 6 5

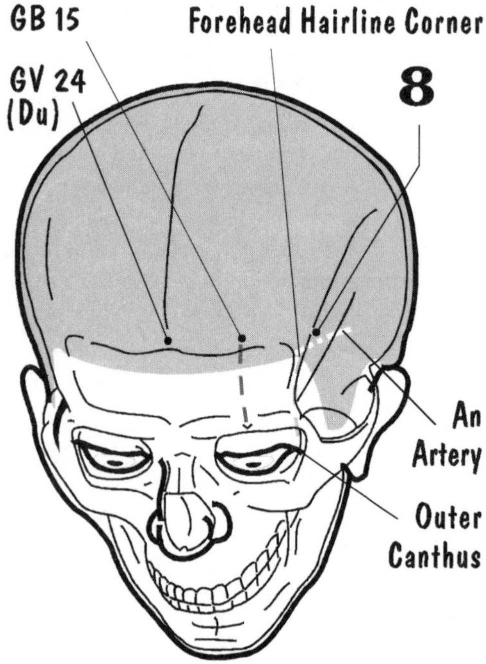

GB 15
Forehead Hairline Corner
GV 24 (Du)
8
An Artery
Outer Canthus

Description:

~ Daying ~ St 5

Location: In the vertical slit on the mandible ridge, anterior to the masseter attachment.

Tips & References: Level with the mandible angle.

☆ Posterior to the facial artery (search for the sensation of pulse).

☆ Search for the slit on the cheek's posterior border when the cheeks are blown up.

☆ Easier to identify the masseter when clenching the teeth.

Note: ....

~ Jiache ~ St 6

Location: In the depression, 1 fingerbreadth (3rd finger) superior and anterior to the mandible angle.

Tips & References: When the teeth are clenched, in the center of the masseter bulge that is formed.

☆ Search for a split in the muscle that can be felt when moving anterior-superiorly from the mandible angle.

Note: ....

~ Xiaguan ~ St 7

Location: When the mouth is closed, in the depression, vertically inferior to the vertical slit on the zygomatic arch inferior border, level with the condylar process.

Tips & References: Level with the tragus inferior notch and GB 2.

☆ Easier to identify the slit while moving posteriorly along the zygomatic arch inferior border.

Basic Feature: Interaction with GB.

Note: ....

~ Touwei ~ St 8

Location: 0.5 cun superior (and lateral) to the forehead hairline corner.

Tips & References: 4.5 cun lateral to front midline and GV(Du) 24*.

☆ Twice of the distance between GV(Du) 24* and GB 15**.

☆ Posterior to the point where there is sensation of pulse.

☆ Normally, the forehead hairline corner is vertically superior to the eye's outer canthus.

☆ The hairline is the borderline between a regular skin tissue and the oilier hair-skin tissue. This borderline can be felt when running the fingernail on the skin.

Basic Feature: Interaction with GB and Yangwei (Ya-L).

Note: ....

* See p. 170.

** See p. 134.

Stomach Meridian

notes:

9
10
11

Hyoid

Laryngeal
Prominence

Thyroid
Cartilage

Common Carotid
Artery

Sternocleidomastoid

Clavicle

Description:

~ Renying ~ St 9

Location: Level with the Adam's apple peak (laryngeal prominance), anterior to the sternocleidomastoid.

Tips & References: The sternocleidomastoid muscle of one side is more distinct when the head is turned to the other side and resisting a pressure applied (e.g. on the chin) from the first side.

☆ On the line starting at the Adam's apple peak (laryngeal prominence) and parallel to the jaw.

☆ Lateral to the thyroid cartilage.

☆ Medial to the common carotid artery, which is located deeply (search for the sensation of pulse).

☆ 1.5 cun / 2 fingerbeadth (2nd and 3rd fingers) lateral to the Adam's apple peak.

☆ When the Adam's apple peak is hard to identify, search for the peak location on the inferior border of the depression formed by the hyoid bone and the thyroid cartilage.

Basic Feature: Sea of Qi. Window to the Sky. Some sources indicate interaction with GB.

Note: ....

~ Shuitu ~ St 10

Location: Anterior to the sternocleidomastoid, level with the midpoint between St 9 and St 11.

Tips & References: St 9, St 10 and St 11 are not on a straight line.

☆ The sternocleidomastoid muscle of one side is more distinct when the head is turned to the other side and resisting a pressure applied (e.g. on the chin) from the first side.

Note: ....

~ Qishe ~ St 11

Location: Between the two heads of the sternocleidomastoid, superior to the clavicle.

Tips & References: Superior to the clavicle medial end.

☆ Vertically inferior to St 9.

☆ The sternocleidomastoid muscle of one side is more distinct when the head is turned to the other side and resisting a pressure applied (e.g. on the chin) from the first side.

Note: ....

Stomach Meridian

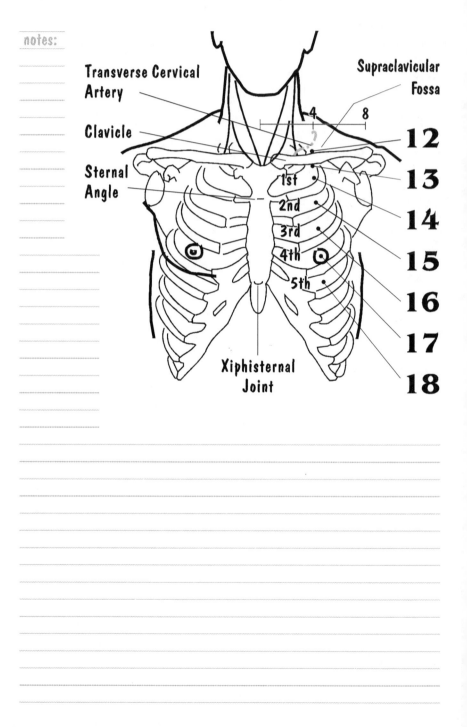

notes:

Transverse Cervical Artery

Supraclavicular Fossa

Clavicle

4   **8**

12

Sternal Angle

1st

13

2nd

14

3rd

4th

15

5th

16

17

Xiphisternal Joint

18

Description:

~ Quepen ~ St 12

Location: Superior to the clavicle, 4 cun lateral to the front midline.

Tips & References: In the supraclavicular fossa.

☆ Vertically superior to the midpoint between the armpit anterior crease (axillary fold) and the front midline.

☆ Inferior to the transverse cervical artery (search for the sensation of pulse).

Basic Feature: Some sources indicate interaction with six Yang meridians and Yinqiao (Yi-H).

Note: ....

~ Qihu ~ St 13

Location: In the gap between the clavicle and the 1st rib, 4 cun lateral to the front midline.

Tips & References: Vertically inferior to St 12.

Note: ....

~ Kufang ~ St 14

Location: In the 1st intercostal, 4 cun lateral to the front midline.

Tips & References: On the line connecting the nipple with St 12.

☆ The 1st intercostal is superior to the 2nd rib which is level with the sternal angle.

Note: ....

~ Wuyi ~ St 15

Location: In the 2nd intercostal, 4 cun lateral to the front midline.

Tips & References: The 2nd intercostal is inferior to the 2nd rib which is level with the sternal angle.

Note: ....

~ Yingchuang ~ St 16

Location: In the 3rd intercostal, 4 cun lateral to the front midline.

Tips & References: The 3rd intercostal is the second space inferior to the 2nd rib which is level with the sternal angle.

Note: ....

~ Ruzhong ~ St 17

Location: In the center of the nipple.

☆ A reference point only: no needling, no pressing, no moxibustion.

Note: ....

~ Rugen ~ St 18

Location: In the 5th intercostal, 4 cun lateral to the front midline.

Tips & References: The 5th intercostal is level with the xiphisternal joint.

☆ In female: on the inferior crease of the breast.

Note: ....

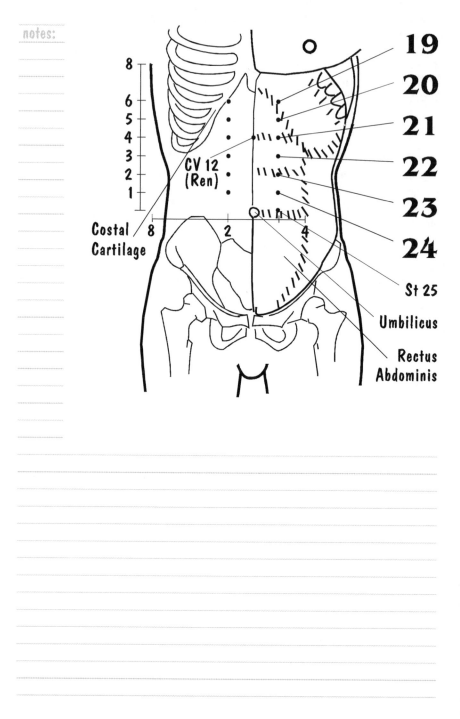

notes:

8
6
5
4
3
2
1

CV 12
(Ren)

Costal
Cartilage 8

2

4

19
20
21
22
23
24

St 25

Umbilicus

Rectus
Abdominis

Description:

Location:
~ Burong ~ St 19
Location: 2 cun lateral to the front midline, level with 6 cun superior to the umbilicus.
Tips & References: On the rectus abdominis (of one side) vertical midline.
☆ Medial to the costal cartilage.
☆ Level with CV(Ren) 14*.
Note: ....

~ Chengman ~ St 20
Location: 2 cun lateral to the front midline, level with 5 cun superior to the umbilicus.
Tips & References: On the rectus abdominis (of one side) vertical midline.
☆ Level with CV(Ren) 13*.
Note: ....

~ Liangmen ~ St 21
Location: 2 cun lateral to the front midline, level with 4 cun superior to the umbilicus.
Tips & References: On the rectus abdominis (of one side) vertical midline.
☆ Level with CV(Ren) 12*.
Note: ....

~ Guanmen ~ St 22
Location: 2 cun lateral to the front midline, level with 3 cun superior to the umbilicus.
Tips & References: On the rectus abdominis (of one side) vertical midline.
☆ Level with CV(Ren) 11*.
Note: ....

~ Taiyi ~ St 23
Location: 2 cun lateral to the front midline, level with 2 cun superior to the umbilicus.
Tips & References: On the rectus abdominis (of one side) vertical midline.
☆ Level with CV(Ren) 10*.
Note: ....

~ Huaroumen ~ St 24
Location: 2 cun lateral to the front midline, level with 1 cun superior to the umbilicus.
Tips & References: On the rectus abdominis (of one side) vertical midline.
☆ Level with CV(Ren) 9*.
Note: ....

* See p. 158.

Stomach Meridian

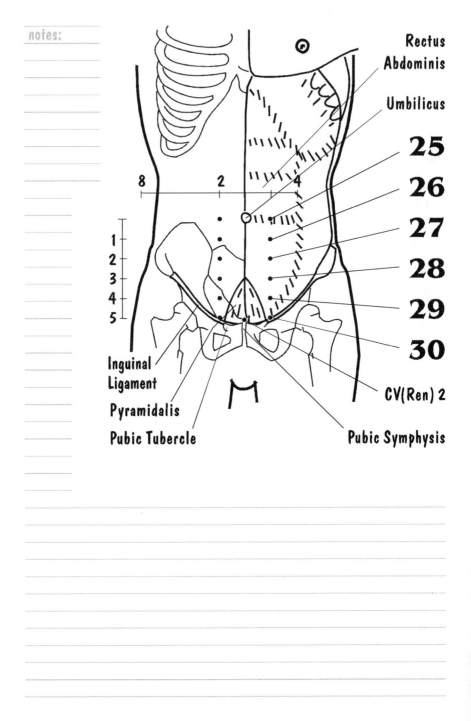

notes:

Rectus
Abdominis

Umbilicus

25

26

27

28

29

30

Inguinal
Ligament

Pyramidalis

Pubic Tubercle

CV(Ren) 2

Pubic Symphysis

Description:

~ Tianshu ~ St 25

Location: 2 cun lateral to the umbilicus center.
Tips & References: On the rectus abdominis (of one side) vertical midline.
☆　Level with CV(Ren) 8*.
Basic Feature: LI front 'Mu' collecting pt..
Note: ....

~ Wailing ~ St 26

Location: 2 cun lateral to the front midline, level with 1 cun inferior to the umbilicus.
Tips & References: On the rectus abdominis (of one side) vertical midline.
☆　Level with CV(Ren) 7*.
Note: ....

~ Daju ~ St 27

Location: 2 cun lateral to the front midline, level with 2 cun inferior to the umbilicus.
Tips & References: On the rectus abdominis (of one side) vertical midline.
☆　Level with CV(Ren) 5*.
Note: ....

~ Shuidao ~ St 28

Location: 2 cun lateral to the front midline, level with 3 cun inferior to the umbilicus.
Tips & References: On the rectus abdominis (of one side) vertical midline.
☆　Level with CV(Ren) 4*.
Note: ....

~ Guilai ~ St 29

Location: 2 cun lateral to the front midline, level with 4 cun inferior to the umbilicus.
Tips & References: Level with CV(Ren) 3*.
Note: ....

~ Qichong ~ St 30

Location: 2 cun lateral to the front midline, level with the pubic symphysis superior border.
Tips & References: Lateral to the pyramidalis.
☆　Superior (and medial) to the inguinal ligament.
☆　Level with CV(Ren) 2*.
☆　Level with 5 cun inferior to the umbilicus.
Basic Feature: Sea of nourishment. Some sources indicate interaction with Chong (Pen.).
Note: ....

* See p. 156.

Stomach Meridian

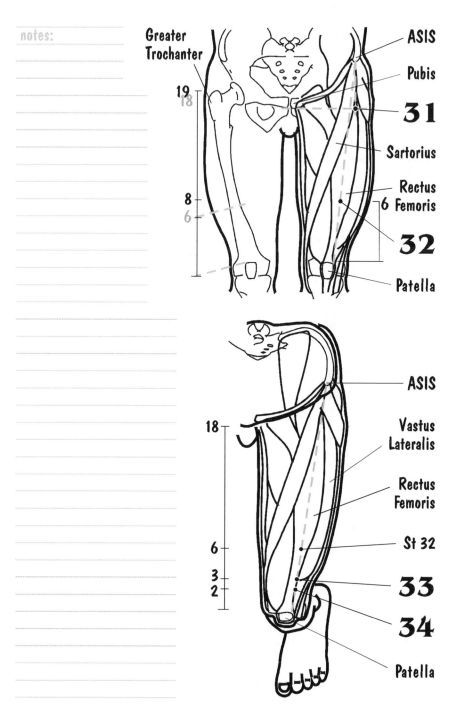

notes:

Greater Trochanter

ASIS

Pubis

31

Sartorius

Rectus Femoris

32

Patella

19
18

8
6

6

ASIS

Vastus Lateralis

Rectus Femoris

St 32

33

34

Patella

18

6
3
2

Description:

~ Biguan ~ St 31

Location: Lateral to the sartorius, level with the pubis inferior border.
Tips & References: Vertically inferior to the ASIS*.
☆ Level with the greater trochanter tip.
☆ <u>On</u> the rectus femoris.
☆ When lying on the back, level with the buttock (gluteal transverse) fold.
☆ In the depression lateral to the sartorius that is formed when the thigh is flexed.
Note: ....

~ Futu ~ St 32

Location: On the line connecting the patella's lateral-superior corner with the
    ASIS*, 6 cun superior to the patella.
Tips & References: 8 cun superior to the knee fold (popliteal crease).
☆ The patella height, which is 2 cun, is a comfortable unit for finding this point.
Note: ....

~ Yinshi ~ St 33

Location: When the leg is bent, on the line connecting the patella lateral-superior
    corner with the ASIS*, 3 cun proximal to the patella.
Tips & References: Between the rectus femoris and the vastus lateralis.
☆ The patella height, which is 2 cun, is a comfortable unit for finding this point.
☆ Easier to identify the point while manipulating the knee.
☆ Search for the second deep depression that can be felt when moving proximally
    from the patella lateral-superior corner.
Note: ....

~ Liangqiu ~ St 34

Location: When the leg is bent, on the line connecting the patella lateral-superior
    corner with the ASIS*, 2 cun proximal to the patella.
Tips & References: Between the rectus femoris and the vastus lateralis.
☆ The patella height, which is 2 cun, is a comfortable unit for finding this point.
☆ Easier to identify the point while manipulating the knee.
☆ Search for the first deep depression that can be felt whan moving proximally
    from the patella lateral-superior corner.
Basic Feature: 'Xi' accumulation pt..
Note: ....

* Anterior Superior Iliac Spine.

Stomach Meridian

notes:

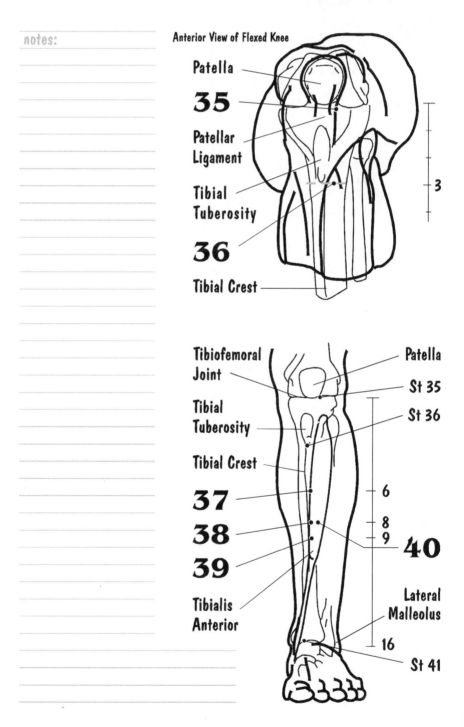

Anterior View of Flexed Knee

Patella

35

Patellar Ligament

Tibial Tuberosity

36

Tibial Crest

3

Tibiofemoral Joint

Patella

St 35

Tibial Tuberosity

St 36

Tibial Crest

37

38

39

6

8
9 **40**

Tibialis Anterior

Lateral Malleolus

16

St 41

Description:

~ Dubi ~ St 35

Location: When the knee is flexed, in the depression, inferior to the patella lateral-inferior corner.

Tips & References: Lateral to the patellar ligament.

☆ Easier to identify the point while manipulating the knee.

Note: ....

~ Zusanli ~ St 36

Location: When the leg is slightly bent, in the depression, level with the tibial tuberosity inferior border, 1 fingerbreadth (3rd finger) lateral to the anterior sharp crest of the tibia.

Tips & References: About 3 cun inferior to the patella's lateral-inferior corner.

☆ Search for the depression at the end of the gap that can be felt when moving superiorly along the lateral border of the tibial shaft.

Basic Feature: 'He' sea, earth, horary pt.. Abdomen command pt.. Sea of nourishment. "Leg, 3 miles."

Note: ....

~ Shangjuxu ~ St 37

Location: 6 cun inferior to the patella, 1 fingerbreadth (3rd finger) lateral to the anterior sharp crest of the tibia*.

☆ About 3 cun inferior to the tibial tuberosity and St 35.

Basic Feature: Sea of blood. LI lower 'He' sea pt..

Note: ....

~ Tiaokou ~ St 38

Location: 8 cun inferior to the patella, 1 fingerbreadth (3rd finger) lateral to the anterior sharp crest of the tibia*.

Tips & References: Midway between St 35 and St 41.

☆ Level with the midpoint between the knee joint and the lateral malleolus peak.

Note: ....

~ Xiajuxu ~ St 39

Location: 9 cun inferior to the patella, 1 fingerbreadth (3rd finger) lateral to the anterior sharp crest of the tibia*.

Basic Feature: SI lower sea point. Sea of blood.

Note: ....

~ Fenglong ~ St 40

Location: 8 cun inferior to the patella, 2 fingerbreadths (2nd and 3rd finger) lateral to the anterior sharp crest of the tibia.

Tips & References: 1 fingerbreadth lateral to St 38.

☆ Level with the midpoint between the knee joint and the lateral malleolus peak.

Basic Feature: 'Luo' connecting pt..

Note: ....

* On the tibialis anterior muscle.

Stomach Meridian

notes:

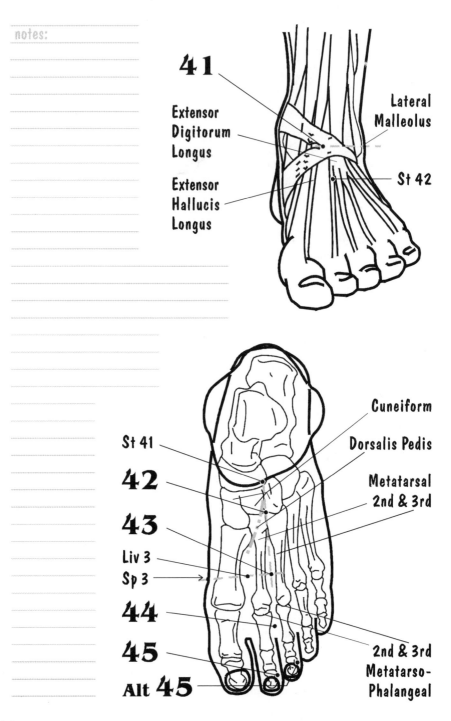

41

Extensor
Digitorum
Longus

Extensor
Hallucis
Longus

Lateral
Malleolus

St 42

St 41

42

43

Liv 3
Sp 3

44

45

Alt **45**

Cuneiform

Dorsalis Pedis

Metatarsal
2nd & 3rd

2nd & 3rd
Metatarso-
Phalangeal

Description:

~ Jiexi ~ St 41

Location: At the ankle joint, between the extensor hallucis longus and extensor digitorum longus tendons.

Tips & References: Easier to identify the tendons when moving the toes.

☆ Level with the lateral malleolus peak.

☆ Search for the extensor hallucis longus that is bigger and extended anteriorly.

Basic Feature: 'Jing' river, fire, tonification pt..

Note: ....

~ Chongyang ~ St 42

Location: In the depression, at the joint of 3 bones: the cuneiform and the 2nd and 3rd metatarsals.

Tips & References: At the highest point on the dorsal aspect of the foot.

☆ On the line connecting St 41 with St 43.

☆ About 2 fingerbreadths distal to St 41.

☆ Lateral to the dorsalis pedis artery (search for the sensation of pulse).

☆ It may be located on either side of the extensor digitorum longus medial slip.

☆ Search for the depression that can be felt when moving proximally from the depression between the two metatarsal bones.

Basic Feature: 'Yuan' source pt..

Note: ....

~ Xiangu ~ St 43

Location: Between the 2nd and 3rd metatarsals, proximal to the bone heads.

Tips & References: Level with Sp 3* and Liv 3**.

☆ Search for the first deep depression that can be felt when moving proximally in the gap between the 2nd and 3rd metatarsophalangeal joints.

Basic Feature: 'Shu' stream, wood pt..

Note: ....

~ Neiting ~ St 44

Location: Between the 2nd and 3rd toes, midway between the web margin and the 2nd metatarsophalangeal joint.

Tips & References: On the borderline between the sole skin and pigmented skin.

Basic Feature: 'Ying' spring, water pt..

Note: ....

~ Lidui ~ St 45

Location: 0.1 cun proximal to the 2nd toenail lateral corner.

Tips & References: Proximal to the nail base.

Alternate Location: 0.1 cun proximal to the 3rd toenail lateral corner.

☆ Proximal to the nail base.

☆ This point is the end of an inner branch of St meridian.

Basic Feature: 'Jing' well, metal, sedation pt..

Note: ....

* See p. 50.
** See p. 150.

~ Points on Foot Taiyin ~
Spleen Meridian

notes:

1

First
Metatarsal

Metatarso-
phalangeal
Joint

First
Proximal
Phalanx

Abductor
Hallucis

4 3 2

Description:

~ Yinbai ~ Sp 1

Location: 0.1 cun proximal to the big toenail medial corner.
Tips & References: Proximal to the nail base.
Basic Feature: 'Jing' well, wood pt.. Interaction with St meridian inner branch.
Note: ....

~ Dadu ~ Sp 2

Location: On the medial aspect of the big toe, inferior and distal to the 1st proximal phalanx bone base.
Tips & References: Distal and inferior to the metatarsophalangeal joint.
☆   On the borderline between the sole skin and pigmented skin.
Basic Feature: 'Ying' spring, fire, tonification pt..
Note: ....

~ Taibai ~ Sp 3

Location: Inferior and proximal to the 1st metatarsal bone head.
Tips & References: Proximal and inferior to the metatarsophalangeal joint.
☆   Between the abductor hallucis tendon and the bone.
☆   On the borderline between the sole skin and pigmented skin.
☆   Search for the end of the gap that can be felt when moving distally along the 1st metatarsal inferior border.
Basic Feature: 'Shu' stream, earth, horary pt.. 'Yuan' source pt..
Note: ....

~ Gongsun ~ Sp 4

Location: Inferior to the 1st metatarsal bone, distal to the bone base.
Tips & References: On the borderline between the sole skin and pigmented skin.
☆   About 1.2 cun proximal to Sp 3.
☆   Between the abductor hallucis tendon and the bone.
☆   Search for the second depression that can be felt when moving proximally from the 1st metatarsal bone head, along the bone's inferior border.
Basic Feature: 'Luo' connecting pt.. Chong (Pen.) opening pt.. Yinwei (Yi-L) coupled pt..
Note: ....

Spleen Meridian

notes:

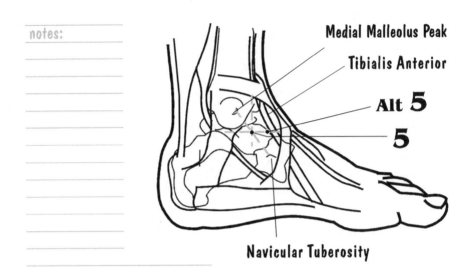

Medial Malleolus Peak

Tibialis Anterior

Alt 5

5

Navicular Tuberosity

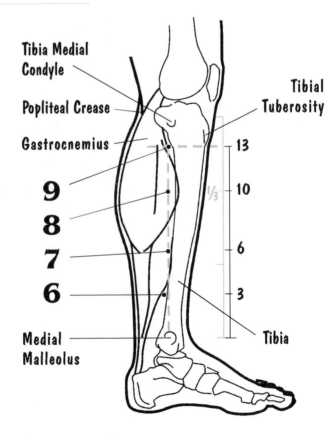

Tibia Medial Condyle

Popliteal Crease

Gastrocnemius

Tibial Tuberosity

9

8

7

6

13

$1/3$ 10

6

3

Medial Malleolus

Tibia

Description:

~ Shangqiu ~ Sp 5

Location: In the depression, level with the medial malleolus inferior border, vertically inferior to the medial malleolus anterior border.

Tips & References: Midway between the navicular tuberosity and the medial malleolus peak.

Alternative Location: In the depression, level with the medial malleolus inferior border, posterior to the tibialis anterior.

☆ 0.5 cun anterior to the meeting of two imaginary lines: the vertical line anterior to the medial malleolus and the horizontal line, inferior to the same malleolus.

Basic Feature: 'Jing' river, metal, sedation point.

Note: ....

~ Sanyinjiao ~ Sp 6

Location: 3 cun superior to the medial malleolus peak, posterior to the tibia.

Tips & References: Search for the point behind the hard tissue, slightly posterior to the area where the bone is clearly felt.

☆ Search for the gap end that can be felt when moving superiorly from the medial malleolus posterior border.

Basic Feature: Interaction with leg's three Yin meridians (K, Liv, Sp) and some sources indicate also interaction with Yinqiao (Yi-H).

Note: ....

~ Lougu ~ Sp 7

Location: 6 cun superior to the medial malleolus peak, posterior to the tibia.

Tips & References: On the line connecting the medial malleolus peak with Sp 9.

☆ 3 cun superior to Sp 6.

☆ Search for the point behind the hard tissue, posterior to the area where the bone is clearly felt.

Note: ....

~ Diji ~ Sp 8

Location: 3 cun inferior to Sp 9, on the line connecting the medial malleolus peak with Sp 9.

Tips & References: In a vertical depression on the muscle.

☆ Level with 1/3 of the distance between the knee posterior crease (popliteal crease) to the medial malleolus peak.

Basic Feature: 'Xi' accumulation pt..

Note: ....

~ Yinlingquan ~ Sp 9

Location: When the leg is straight, in the depression, vertically inferior to the tibial medial condyle, level with the inferior border of the tibial tuberosity.

Tips & References: Anterior to the gastrocnemius.

☆ Search for the depression that can be felt when moving proximally along the tibia posterior border.

Basic Feature: 'He' sea, water pt..

Note: ....

Spleen Meridian

notes:

10

Patella

Sp 11

Rectus Femoris

Vastus Medialis

2 cun

Sp 12

Gracilis

Sartorius

Femoral
Artery

18

11

6

Sp 10

Medial Condyle

Description:

~ Xuehai ~ Sp 10

Location: When the leg is flexed, in the depression, 2 cun proximal to the patella medial-superior corner.

Tips & References: The depression can be felt in the center of the bulge that is formed when the knee is flexed.

☆   Medial to the vastus medialis midline.

☆   The patella height, which is 2 cun, is a comfortable unit for finding this point.

☆   Search for a split in the muscle that can be felt when moving proximally from the patella corner.

Basic Feature: Point of blood treatment.

Note: ....

~ Jimen ~ Sp 11

Location: On the line connecting Sp 10 and Sp 12, 6 cun proximal to Sp 10.

Tips & References: Between the sartorius and the gracilis muscles.

☆   Search for the sensation of pulse of femoral artery.

Note: ....

Spleen Meridian

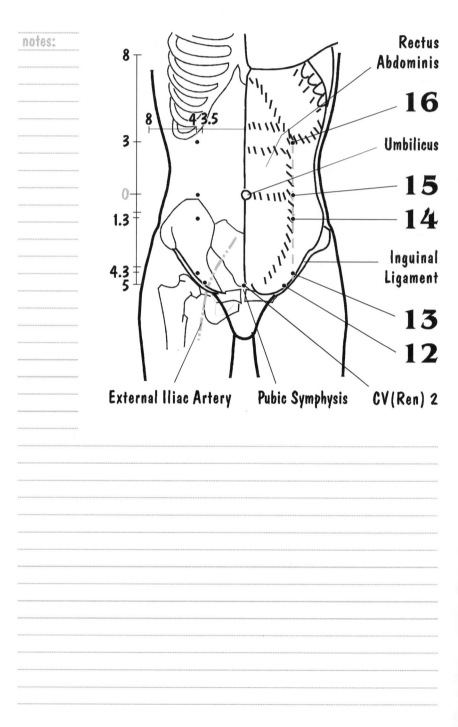

notes:

Rectus
Abdominis

16

Umbilicus

15

14

Inguinal
Ligament

13

12

External Iliac Artery   Pubic Symphysis   CV(Ren) 2

Description:

~ Chongmen ~ Sp 12

Location: 3.5 cun lateral to front midline, superior to the inguinal ligament.

Tips & References: Level with the pubic symphysis superior border and CV(Ren) 2*.

☆ Lateral to the external iliac artery (search for the sensation of pulse).

Basic Feature: Interaction with Liv.

Note: ....

~ Fushe ~ Sp 13

Location: 4 cun lateral to front midline, superior to the inguinal ligament.

Tips & References: Lateral and 0.7 cun superior to Sp 12.

☆ Lateral to the rectus abdominis.

☆ Search for the first deep depression that can be felt when moving laterally (and superior) from Sp 12 along the inguinal ligament superior border.

Basic Feature: Interaction with Liv and Yinwei (Yi-L).

Note: ....

~ Fujie ~ Sp 14

Location: 4 cun lateral to the front midline, level with 1.3 cun inferior to the umbilicus.

Tips & References: Lateral to the rectus abdominis.

☆ 3 cun (1 handbreadth) superior to Sp 13.

☆ 1.3 cun inferior to Sp 15.

Note: ....

~ Daheng ~ Sp 15

Location: 4 cun lateral to the umbilicus center.

Tips & References: Lateral to the rectus abdominis.

☆ Level with CV(Ren) 8*.

Basic Feature: Interaction with Yinwei (Yi-L).

Note: ....

~ Fuai ~ Sp 16

Location: 4 cun lateral to the front midline, level with 3 cun (1 handbreadth) superior to the umbilicus.

Tips & References: Lateral to the rectus abdominis.

☆ 3 cun superior to Sp 15.

☆ Level with CV(Ren) 11**.

Basic Feature: Interaction with Yinwei (Yi-L).

Note: ....

* See p. 156.
** See p. 158.

Spleen Meridian

notes:

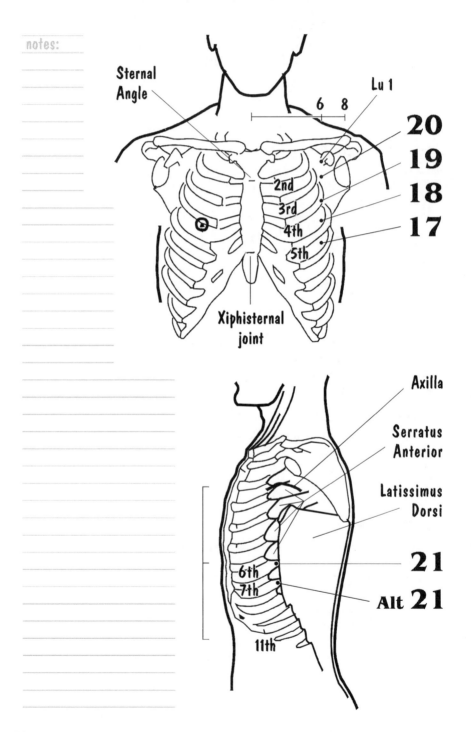

Sternal Angle

Lu 1

6 8

20
19
18
17

2nd
3rd
4th
5th

Xiphisternal joint

Axilla

Serratus Anterior

Latissimus Dorsi

21

Alt 21

6th
7th

11th

Description:

~ Shidou ~ Sp 17

Location: In the 5th intercostal, 6 cun lateral to the front midline.
Tips & References: The 5th intercostal medial end is level with the xiphisternal joint.
Note: ....

~ Tianxi ~ Sp 18

Location: In the 4th intercostal, 6 cun lateral to the front midline.
Tips & References: Male's nipple is level with the 4th intercostal.
☆ In males, the point is located 2 cun lateral to the nipple.
Note: ....

~ Xiongxiang ~ Sp 19

Location: In the 3rd intercostal, 6 cun lateral to the front midline.
Tips & References: The 3rd intercostal is the second space inferior to the 2nd rib which is level with the sternal angle.
Note: ....

~ Zhourong ~ Sp 20

Location: In the 2nd intercostal, 6 cun lateral to the front midline.
Tips & References: Vertically inferior to Lu 1* (follow the body landmarks).
☆ The 2nd intercostal is inferior to the 2nd rib which is level with the sternal angle.
Note: ....

~ Dabao ~ Sp 21

Location: In the 6th intercostal, inferior to the armpit (axilla) center.
Tips & References: Anterior to the latissimus dorsi muscle.
☆ Midpoint between the axilla apex and the 11th rib anterior free end.
☆ When the arm is horizontal (abduction), 6 cun inferior to the axilla.
Alternative Location: In the 7th intercostal, inferior to the armpit center.
☆ Anterior to the latissimus dorsi.
Basic Feature: Interaction with all connecting meridians.
Note: ....

* See p. 16.

Heart Meridian

notes:

Axillary
Artery

1

Pectoralis major   Latissimus Dorsi

Biceps Brachii   **2** **3**

Brachialis

H 1

9   3

Cubital Crease   Medial
Epicondyle

Description:

~ Jiquan ~ H 1

Location: When the arm is raised (abduction), in the center of the armpit (axilla), medial to the axillary artery.

Tips & References: Search for the sensation of pulse.

☆ At the deepest point between the front and back muscles that define the armpit.

☆ At the axillary depression superior part.

Note: ....

~ Qingling ~ H 2

Location: When the elbow is flexed, 3 cun proximal to the elbow (cubital) crease medial end, medial to the biceps brachii.

Tips & References: On the line connecting H 1 with H 3.

☆ Between the biceps brachii muscle and the brachialis muscle.

Note: ....

~ Shaohai ~ H 3

Location: When the elbow is bent at a right angle, between the medial epicondyle and the cubital crease medial end.

Tips & References: When pressing this point, tickling sensation might be felt in the little finger.

☆ Search for the gap between the soft and hard tissues.

Basic Feature: 'He' sea, water pt..

Note: ....

Heart Meridian

notes:

12

Carpal Crease

Flexor
Carpi
Ulnaris

1.5
1
0.5

4

5

6

H 7

Description:

~ Lingdao ~ H 4

Location: When the arm is straight and the palm faces the anterior (supination), 1.5 cun proximal to the carpal (wrist) crease, radial to the flexor carpi ulnaris tendon.

Basic Feature: 'Jing' river, metal pt..

Note: ....

~ Tongli ~ H 5

Location: When the arm is straight and the palm faces the anterior (supination), 1 cun proximal to the carpal (wrist) crease, radial to the flexor carpi ulnaris tendon.

Basic Feature: 'Luo' connecting pt..

Note: ....

~ Yinxi ~ H 6

Location: When the arm is straight and the palm faces the anterior (supination), 0.5 cun proximal to the carpal (wrist) crease, radial to the flexor carpi ulnaris tendon.

Basic Feature: 'Xi' accumulation pt..

Note: ....

Heart Meridian

notes:

8

4th & 5th
Metacarpal

Pisiform

7

Flexor
Carpi Ulnaris

9

H 8

Description:

~ Shenmen ~ H 7

Location: When the arm is straight and the palm faces the anterior (supination), in the carpal (wrist) joint, radial to the flexor carpi ulnaris tendon.

Tips & References: At the ulnar end of the carpal (wrist) crease.

☆ Proximal to pisiform radial corner.

☆ Search for the gap end that can be felt when moving distally along the flexor carpi ulnaris tendon radial border.

Basic Feature: 'Shu' stream, earth, sedation pt.. 'Yuan' source pt..

Note: ....

~ Shaofu ~ H 8

Location: In the depression, between the 4th and 5th metacarpal bones, about 0.3 cun proximal to the bone heads.

Tips & References: When fisting the hand, where the tip of the little finger rests.

☆ Between the two typical palm transverse creases.

Basic Feature: 'Ying' spring, fire, horary pt..

Note: ....

~ Shaochong ~ H 9

Location: 0.1 cun proximal to the little fingernail radial corner.

Tips & References: Proximal to the nail base.

Basic Feature: 'Jing' well, wood, tonification pt..

Note: ....

Small Intestine Meridian

notes:

5th Proximal Phalanx

Metacarpophalangeal Joint

5th Metacarpal

Pisiform Triquetral

Ulna Styloid Process

2 3 4 5

Description:

~ Shaoze ~ SI 1

Location: 0.1 cun proximal to the little fingernail ulnar corner.
Tips & References: Proximal to the nail base.
Basic Feature: 'Jing' well, metal pt..
Note: ....

~ Qiangu ~ SI 2

Location: When the hand is slightly flexed, on the ulnar aspect of the hand, distal to the 5th proximal phalanx bone base, palmar to the bone neck.
Tips & References: On the borderline between the palm skin and pigmented skin.
☆ Between the bone and a muscle.
☆ Distal to the metacarpophalangeal joint.
Basic Feature: 'Ying' spring, water pt..
Note: ....

~ Houxi ~ SI 3

Location: When the hand is slightly flexed, on the ulnar aspect of the hand, proximal to the 5th metacarpal bone head, palmar to the bone neck.
Tips & References: On the borderline between the palm skin and pigmented skin.
☆ Between the bone and a muscle.
☆ At the ulnar end of the palm distal crease.
☆ Proximal to the metacarpophalangeal joint.
Basic Feature: 'Shu' stream, wood, tonification pt.. GV(Du) opening pt.. Yangqiao (Ya-H) coupled pt..
Note: ....

~ Wangu ~ SI 4

Location: In the depression, at the meeting point of three bones: the triquetral, the pisiform and the base of the 5th metacarpal.
Basic Feature: 'Yuan' source pt..
Note: ....

~ Yanggu ~ SI 5

Location: At the meeting point of three bones: the triquetral, the pisiform and the ulna styloid process.
Tips & References: At the ulnar end of the wrist crease.
Basic Feature: 'Jing' river, fire, horary pt..
Note: ....

~ Points on Hand Taiyang ~
Small Intestine Meridian

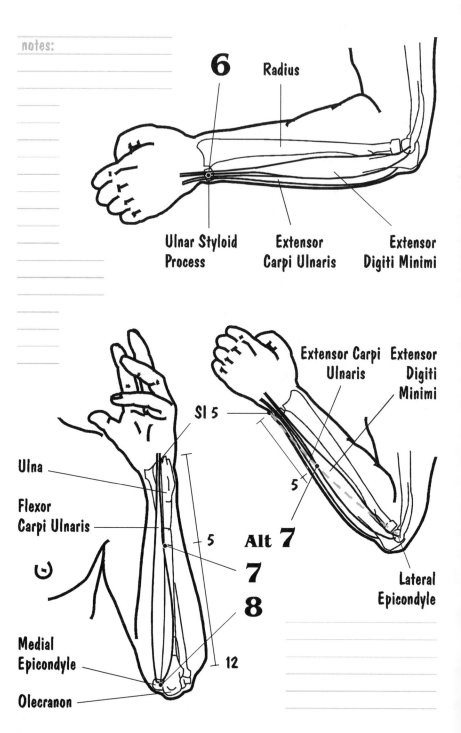

6

Radius

Ulnar Styloid
Process

Extensor
Carpi Ulnaris

Extensor
Digiti Minimi

Extensor Carpi
Ulnaris

Extensor
Digiti
Minimi

SI 5

Ulna

Flexor
Carpi Ulnaris

5

Alt **7**

7

8

Medial
Epicondyle

Olecranon

5

12

Lateral
Epicondyle

~ Acupoint Location Guide ~

Description:

~ Yanglao ~ SI 6

Location: When the palm rests on the breast, in the depression, radial to the ulna styloid tip.

Tips & References: Between the extensor carpi ulnaris and the extensor digiti minimi muscles.

☆   About 1 cun proximal to the wrist joint and crease.

☆   The point is in the slit that disappears when turning the palm inward or outward (pronation or extreme supination).

Basic Feature: 'Xi' accumulation pt..

Note: ....

~ Zhizheng ~ SI 7

Location: When the elbow is flexed and the palm faces the anterior (pronation), on the line connecting SI 5 with SI 8, 5 cun proximal to SI 5.

Tips & References: Between the flexor carpi ulnaris and the ulna.

☆   On the palmar aspect of the ulna.

☆   Search for a horizontal slit on the ulna.

Alternative Location: When the palm rests on the breast, on the line connecting SI 5 with the lateral epicondyle, 5 cun proximal to the wrist crease.

☆   Between the extensor carpi ulnaris and the extensor digiti minimi muscles.

☆   This alternative location is related to a revisionist approach which places the point on the Yang side of the arm since it is a Yang meridian.

Basic Feature: 'Luo' connecting pt..

Note: ....

~ Xiaohai ~ SI 8

Location: When the elbow is flexed and the palm faces the body midline, in the pit, midpoint between the olecranon peak and the medial epicondyle.

Tips & References: Between the flexor carpi ulnaris and the ulna.

Basic Feature: 'He' sea, earth, sedation pt..

Note: ....

Small Intestine Meridian

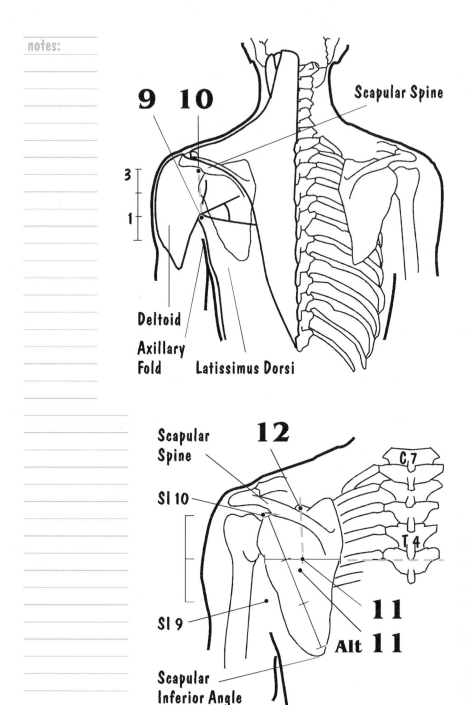

9 10

Scapular Spine

3

1

Deltoid

Axillary
Fold

Latissimus Dorsi

Scapular
Spine

12

C 7

SI 10

T 4

11

SI 9

Alt 11

Scapular
Inferior Angle

Description:

~ Jianzhen ~ SI 9

Location: When the arm lies straight alongside the body (adduction), in the depression, 1 cun superior to the armpit crease (axillary fold) posterior end.

Tips & References: Inferior (and medial) to the deltoid.

☆ On the latissimus dorsi muscle.

☆ Search for the deep depression that can be felt inferior to a meeting of two muscles.

Note: ....

~ Naoshu ~ SI 10

Location: When the arm lies straight alongside the body (adduction), vertically superior to the armpit crease (axillary fold) posterior end, inferior to the scapular spine.

Tips & References: Vertically superior to SI 9.

☆ Search for the point in a superior movement from the armpit crease, along the body land marks. The point might be located slightly lateral to the vertical line.

☆ Search for the point at the depression that can be felt when moving laterally from the scapula medial side, along the spine's inferior border.

Basic Feature: Interaction with Yangwei (Ya-L) and Yangqiao (Ya-H) and many sources indicate also interaction with UB.

Note: ....

~ Tianzong ~ SI 11

Location: Level with 1/3 of the distance between the scapular spine inferior border (e.g. SI 10) and the scapular edge (inferior angle), midway between the scapula's two sides (medial and lateral).

Tips & References: First check the vertical line (between the scapular spine inferior border and the scapular inferior edge).

☆ Level with T4 spinous process.

☆ Normally, level with the midpoint between SI 9 and SI 10.

Alternative Location: The center of the infra scapular fossa, midway in each direction.

Note: ....

~ Bingfeng ~ SI 12

Location: On the scapular spine superior border, vertically superior to SI 11.

Tips & References: In the center of the suprascapular fossa.

☆ In the notch that is formed when lifting the hand.

☆ Search for the point in a superior movement from SI 11, along the body land marks. The point might be located slightly lateral to the vertical line.

☆ Search for the point in the deepest depression that can be felt when moving laterally from the medial part of the scapular spine along the spine's superior border.

Basic Feature: Interaction point with LI , TW(SJ) and GB.

Note: ....

Small Intestine Meridian

notes:

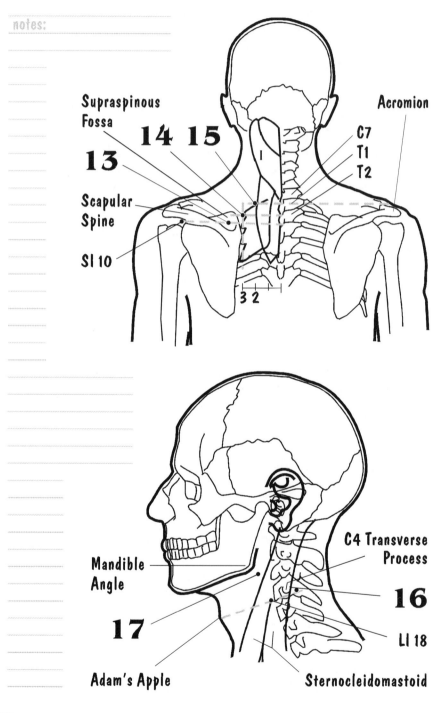

Supraspinous Fossa

14 15

13

Scapular Spine

SI 10

Acromion

C7
T1
T2

3 2

Mandible Angle

17

Adam's Apple

C4 Transverse Process

16

LI 18

Sternocleidomastoid

Description:

~ Quyuan ~ SI 13

Location: In the depression, in the supraspinous fossa medial side.

Tips & References: Midway between SI 10 and T2 spinous process.

☆ The distance between SI 13 & 14 is equal to the distance between SI 14 & 15.

☆ Search for the first deep depression that can be felt when moving (about 1.3 cun) lateral-superiorly from the scapular spine medial end.

☆ The depression can be felt also in a medial search along the scapular spine superior border.

Note: ....

~ Jianwaishu ~ SI 14

Location: 3 cun lateral to T1 spinous process inferior border.

Tips & References: Level with GV(Du) 13***.

☆ When the arm lies straight alongside the body (adduction), vertically superior to the scapular spine medial end.

☆ T1 spinous process is the most extended process on the neck base. Search for the second process that can be felt when moving inferiorly along the neck midline (when the head is anteriorly dropped, T1 is the first spinous process to be felt).

Note: ....

~ Jianzhongshu ~ SI 15

Location: 2 cun lateral to C7 spinous process inferior border.

Tips & References: Level with GV(Du) 14***. Normally, level with the acromion.

☆ Lateral to a hard tissue.

☆ Search for the first spinous process that can be felt when moving inferiorly along the neck midline (when the head is anteriorly dropped, C7 spinous process disappears).

Note: ....

~ Tianchuang ~ SI 16

Location: Level with the Adam's apple peak (laryngeal prominence), posterior to the sternocleidomastoid*.

Tips & References: Posterior (and superior) to LI 18**.

☆ On the line starting at the Adam's apple peak and parallel to the jaw.

☆ Lateral to C4 transverse process.

☆ When the adam's apple peak is hard to identify search for the peak location inferior to the depression formed by the hyoid bone and the thyroid cartilage**.

Basic Feature: Window to the Sky.

Note: ....

~ Tianrong ~ SI 17

Location: Between the mandible angle and the sternocleidomastoid*.

Basic Feature: Window to the Sky.

Note: ....

* The sternocleidomastoid muscle of one side is more distinct when the head is turned to the other side and resisting a pressure applied from the first side.

** See p. 30.   *** See p. 166.

~ Points on Hand Taiyang ~

Small Intestine Meridian

notes:

Outer Canthus
Zygomatic Arch
18
LI 20

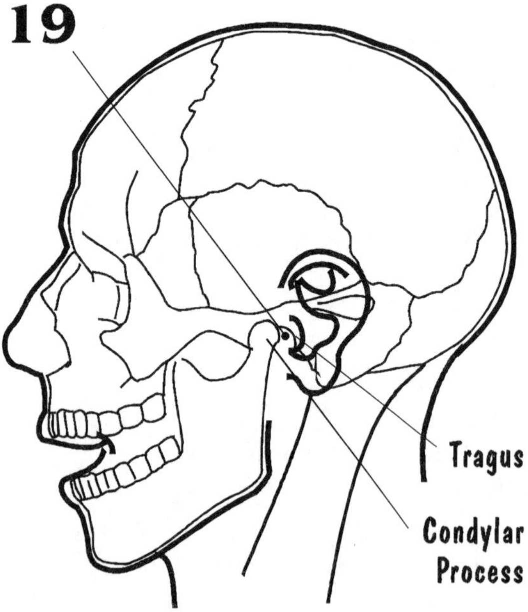

19
Tragus
Condylar Process

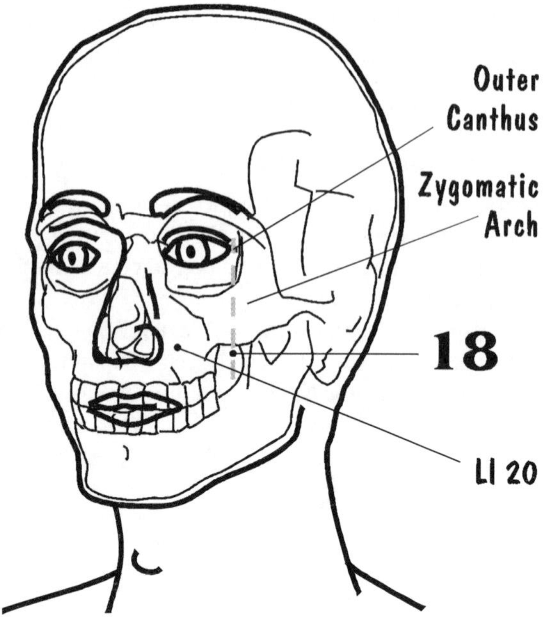

Description:

~ Quanliao ~ SI 18

Location: Vertically inferior to the outer canthus, inferior to the slit on the zygomatic arch inferior border.
Tips & References: Level with LI 20*.
Basic Feature: Interaction with TW(SJ).
Note: ....

~ Tinggong ~ SI 19

Location: When the mouth is open, level with the tragus center, between the tragus and the condylar process.
Tips & References: When the finger touches the condylar process, in the depression that is formed under the finger tip when opening the mouth.
Basic Feature: Interaction with TW(SJ) and GB.
Note: ....

* See p. 30.

Urinary Bladder Meridian

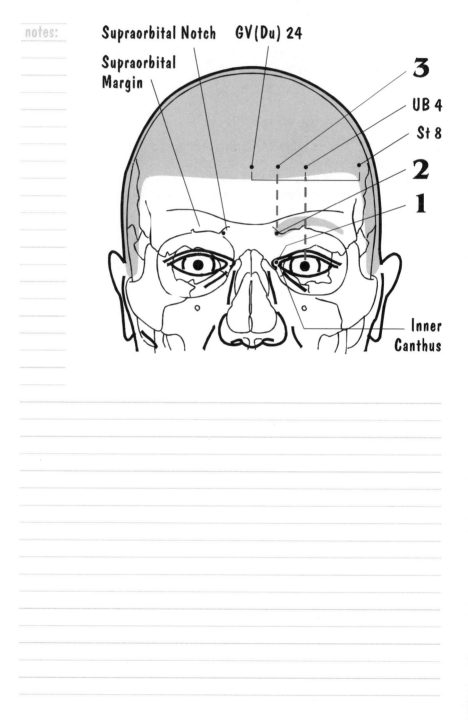

notes:

Supraorbital Notch   GV(Du) 24

Supraorbital
Margin

3

UB 4

St 8

2

1

Inner
Canthus

Description:

~ Jingming ~ UB 1

Location: 0.1 cun superior and medial to the inner canthus.

Tips & References: In the eyelid crease medial part.

Basic Feature: Interaction with St, SI, Yangqiao (Ya-H) and some sources indicate also interaction with Yinqiao (Yi-H), TW(SJ), GB, and GV(Du).

Note: ....

~ Zanzhu ~ UB 2

Location: On the eyebrow medial end, at the supraorbital notch center.

Tips & References: On the supraorbital margin.

☆ Vertically superior to the inner canthus and UB 1.

Note: ....

~ Meichong ~ UB 3

Location: 0.5 cun superior to the forehead hairline, vertically superior to the eyebrow medial end.

Tips & References: Vertically superior to UB 2.

☆ Midpoint between GV(Du) 24* and UB 4.

☆ 0.75 cun lateral to the front midline.

☆ The hairline is the borderline between a regular skin tissue and the oilier hair-skin tissue. This borderline can be felt when running the fingernail on the skin.

Note: ....

* See p. 170.

Urinary Bladder Meridian

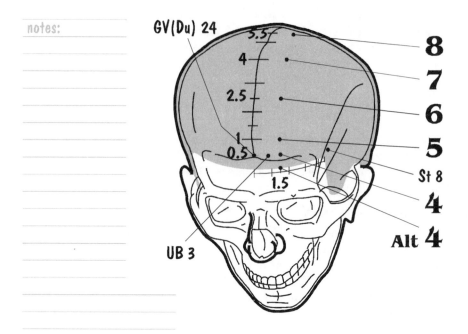

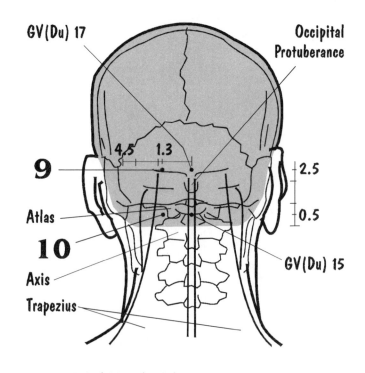

~ Acupoint Location Guide ~

Description:

Location:

~ Quchai ~ UB 4

Location: 0.5 cun superior to the forehead hairline, 1.5 cun lateral to the head midline.

Alternative Location: On the forehead hairline, 1.5 cun lateral to the head midline.

Tips & References: 1/3 of the distance between GV(Du) 24* and St 8**.

Note: ....

~ Wuchu ~ UB 5

Location: 1 cun superior to the forehead hairline, 1.5 cun lateral to the head midline.

Note: ....

~ Chengguang ~ UB 6

Location: 2.5 cun posterior to the forehead hairline, 1.5 cun lateral to the head midline.

Tips & References: 1.5 cun posterior to UB 5.

Note: ....

~ Tongtian ~ UB 7

Location: 4 cun posterior to the forehead hairline, 1.5 cun lateral to the head midline.

Tips & References: 1.5 cun posterior to UB 6.

Note: ....

~ Luoque ~ UB 8

Location: 5.5 cun posterior to the forehead hairline, 1.5 cun lateral to the head midline.

Tips & References: 1.5 cun posterior to UB 7.

Note: ....

~ Yuzhen ~ UB 9

Location: 1.3 cun lateral to head midline, level with the external occipital protuberance superior border.

Tips & References: Level with 2.5 cun superior to the neck hairline.

☆   Level with GV(Du) 17***.

Note: ....

~ Tianzhu ~ UB 10

Location: Level with 0.5 cun inferior to the external occipital protuberance, 1.3 cun lateral to back midline.

Tips & References: On the trapezius lateral aspect.

☆   Inferior to the Atlas/C1 spinous process inferior edge (hard to palpate)

☆   Level with 0.5 cun superior to the neck hairline and GV(Du) 15***.

Basic Feature: Sea of Qi. Window to the Sky.

Note: ....

* See p. 170.   ** See p. 34.   *** See p. 168.

Urinary Bladder Meridian

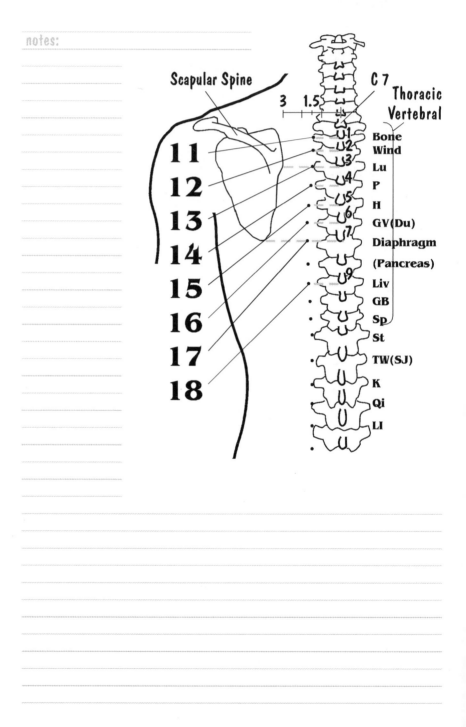

notes:

Scapular Spine

3 1.5

C 7

Thoracic
Vertebral

Bone
Wind
Lu
P
H
GV(Du)
Diaphragm
(Pancreas)
Liv
GB
Sp
St
TW(SJ)
K
Qi
LI

11
12
13
14
15
16
17
18

Description:

~ Dazhu ~ UB 11
Location: 1.5 cun lateral to T1 spinous process inferior edge.
Tips & References: Level with GV(Du) 13*.
☆ Search for the second, most extended process on the neck, that can be felt when moving inferiorly along the neck midline (with the head straight).
Basic Feature: Bones 'Hui' gathering pt.. Sea of blood. Interaction with SI, TW(SJ), GB and some sources indicate also interaction with GV(Du).
Note: ....

~ Fengmen ~ UB 12
Location: 1.5 cun lateral to T2 spinous process inferior edge.
Basic Feature: Interaction with GV(Du).
Note: ....

~ Feishu ~ UB 13
Location: 1.5 cun lateral to T3 spinous process inferior edge.
Tips & References: Level with the scapular spine medial end and GV(Du) 12*.
Basic Feature: Lu back 'Shu' transporting pt..
Note: ....

~ Jueyinshu ~ UB 14
Location: 1.5 cun lateral to T4 spinous process inferior edge.
Basic Feature: P back 'Shu' transporting pt..
Note: ....

~ Xinshu ~ UB 15
Location: 1.5 cun lateral to T5 spinous process inferior edge.
Tips & References: Level with GV(Du) 11*.
Basic Feature: H back 'Shu' transporting pt..
Note: ....

~ Dushu ~ UB 16
Location: 1.5 cun lateral to T6 spinous process inferior edge.
Tips & References: Level with GV(Du) 10*.
Basic Feature: GV(Du) back 'Shu' transporting pt..
Note: ....

~ Geshu ~ UB 17
Location: 1.5 cun lateral to T7 spinous process inferior edge.
Tips & References: Level with the scapular inferior edge and GV(Du) 9*.
Basic Feature: Diaphragm back 'Shu' transporting pt.. Blood 'Hui' gathering pt..
Note: ....

~ Ganshu ~ UB 18
Location: 1.5 cun lateral to T9 spinous process inferior edge.
Tips & References: Level with GV(Du) 8*.
Basic Feature: Liv back 'Shu' transporting pt..
Note: ....

* See p. 166.

Urinary Bladder Meridian

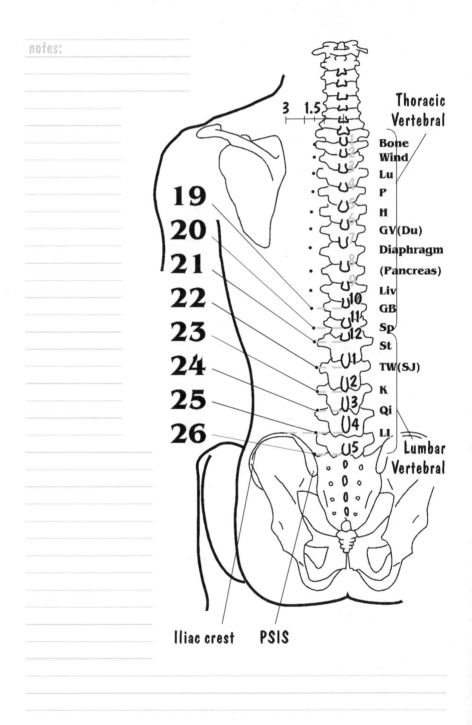

notes:

Thoracic
Vertebral

3   1.5

Bone
Wind
Lu
P
H
GV(Du)
Diaphragm
(Pancreas)
Liv
GB
Sp
St
TW(SJ)
K
Qi
LI

Lumbar
Vertebral

19
20
21
22
23
24
25
26

Iliac crest   PSIS

Description:

~ Danshu ~ UB 19

Location: 1.5 cun lateral to T10 spinous process inferior edge.
Basic Feature: GB back 'Shu' transporting pt..
Note: ....

~ Pishu ~ UB 20

Location: 1.5 cun lateral to T11 spinous process inferior edge.
Tips & References: Level with GV(Du) 6*.
Basic Feature: Sp back 'Shu' transporting pt..
Note: ....

~ Weishu ~ UB 21

Location: 1.5 cun lateral to T12 spinous process inferior edge.
Basic Feature: St back 'Shu' transporting pt..
Note: ....

~ Sanjiaoshu ~ UB 22

Location: 1.5 cun lateral to L1 spinous process inferior edge.
Tips & References: Level with GV(Du) 5**.
Basic Feature: TW(SJ) back 'Shu' transporting pt..
Note: ....

~ Shenshu ~ UB 23

Location: 1.5 cun lateral to L2 spinous process inferior edge.
Tips & References: Level with the 12th rib free end and with GV(Du) 4**.
Basic Feature: K back 'Shu' transporting pt..
Note: ....

~ Qihaishu ~ UB 24

Location: 1.5 cun lateral to L3 spinous process inferior edge.
Tips & References: Vertically superior to the PSIS*** medial border.
Note: ....

~ Dachangshu ~ UB 25

Location: 1.5 cun lateral to L4 spinous process inferior edge.
Tips & References: Level with GV(Du) 3**.
☆ Vertically superior to the PSIS medial border.
☆ Normally, level with the iliac superior crest.
Basic Feature: LI back 'Shu' transporting pt..
Note: ....

~ Guanyuanshu ~ UB 26

Location: 1.5 cun lateral to L5 spinous process inferior edge.
Tips & References: Vertically superior to the PSIS medial border.
Basic Feature: Essence gate. Back 'Shu' transporting pt..
Note: ....

* See p. 166.   ** See p. 164.   *** Posterior Superior Iliac Spine.

Urinary Bladder Meridian

notes:

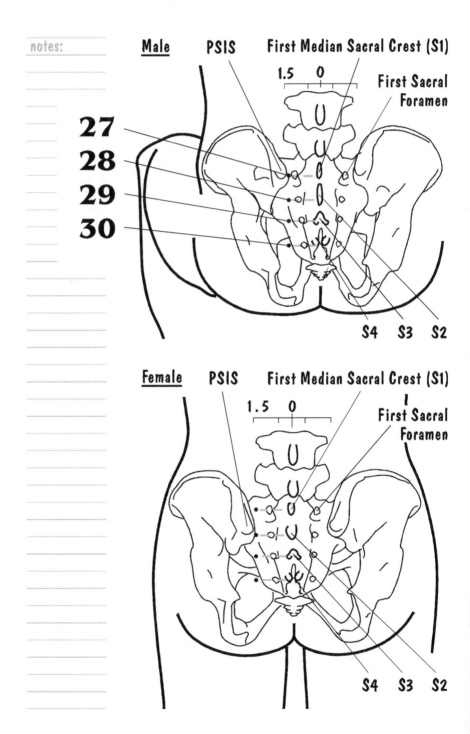

Male PSIS First Median Sacral Crest (S1)

1.5 0 First Sacral Foramen

27
28
29
30

S4 S3 S2

Female PSIS First Median Sacral Crest (S1)

1.5 0 First Sacral Foramen

S4 S3 S2

Description:

~ Xiaochangshu ~ UB 27

Location: Level with the 1st sacral foramen, 1.5 cun lateral to the back midline.
Tips & References: Medial to the PSIS*.
☆　Search for the depression that can be felt when moving laterally from S1 (the first median sacral crest) inferior part.
Basic Feature: SI back 'Shu' transporting pt..
Note: ....

~ Pangguangshu ~ UB 28

Location: Level with the 2nd sacral foramen, 1.5 cun lateral to the back midline.
Tips & References: In male, the point is inferior to the PSIS* medial border. In female, the point is medial to the PSIS*.
☆　Search for the depression that can be felt when moving laterally from S2 (the 2nd median sacral crest) inferior part.
Basic Feature: UB back 'Shu' transporting pt..
Note: ....

~ Zhonglushu ~ UB 29

Location: Level with the 3rd sacral foramen, 1.5 cun lateral to the back midline.
Tips & References: Vertically inferior to the PSIS* medial border.
☆　Easier to identify the anatomical structure when sitting.
☆　Search for the depression that can be felt when moving laterally from S3 (the 3rd median sacral crest) inferior part.
Note: ....

~ Baihuanshu ~ UB 30

Location: Level with the 4th sacral foramen, 1.5 cun lateral to the back midline.
Tips & References: Vertically inferior to the PSIS* medial border.
☆　Easier to identify the anatomical structure when sitting.
☆　Search for the depression that can be felt when moving laterally from S4 (the 4th median sacral crest) inferior part.
Note: ....

* Posterior Superior Iliac Spine.

Urinary Bladder Meridian

notes:

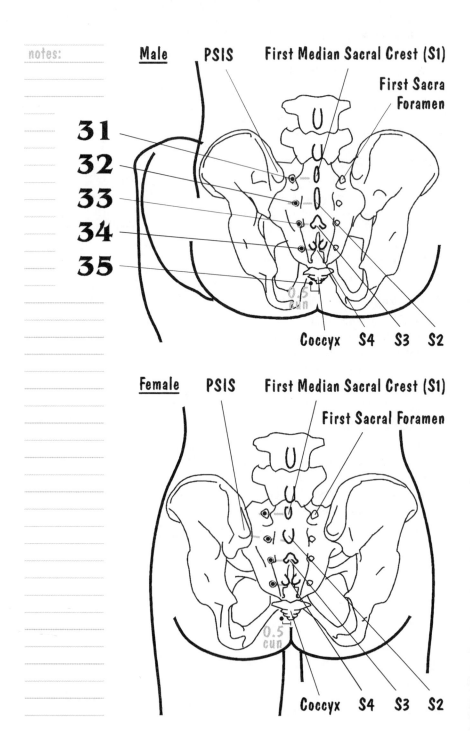

Male   PSIS   First Median Sacral Crest (S1)

First Sacra
Foramen

31
32
33
34
35

0.5
cun

Coccyx S4 S3 S2

Female   PSIS   First Median Sacral Crest (S1)

First Sacral Foramen

0.5
cun

Coccyx S4 S3 S2

Description:

~ Shangliao ~ UB 31

Location: In the 1st sacral foramen.
Tips & References: About midway between the PSIS and the back midline.
☆   Male's 1st sacral foramen is normally slightly lateral to the midpoint between the PSIS and the back midline, female's 1st sacral foramen is normally slightly superior to this midpoint.
☆   Level with S1 (the 1st median sacral crest) inferior part.
Note: ....

~ Ciliao ~ UB 32

Location: In the 2nd sacral foramen.
Tips & References: Inferior and slightly medial to UB 31.
☆   Level with S2 (the 2nd median sacral crest) inferior part.
Note: ....

~ Zhongliao ~ UB 33

Location: In the 3rd sacral foramen.
Tips & References: Inferior and slightly medial to UB 32.
☆   Level with S3 (the 3rd median sacral crest) inferior part.
Basic Feature: Some sources indicate interaction with GB and Liv.
Note: ....

~ Xialiao ~ UB 34

Location: In the 4th sacral foramen.
Tips & References: Inferior and slightly medial to UB 33.
☆   Level with S4 (the 4th median sacral crest) inferior part.
Note: ....

~ Huiyang ~ UB 35

Location: 0.5 cun lateral to coccyx tip.
Note: ....

Urinary Bladder Meridian

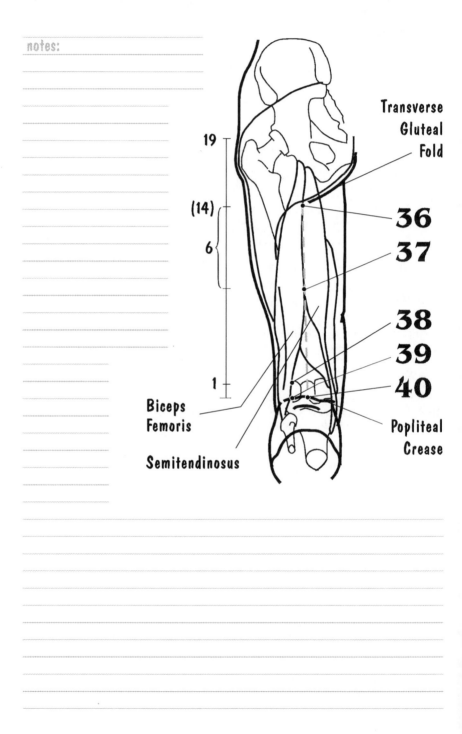

notes:

Transverse
Gluteal
Fold

19

(14)

6

36

37

38

39

40

1

Biceps
Femoris

Semitendinosus

Popliteal
Crease

Description:

~ Chengfu ~ UB 36

Location: When lying on the belly (prone position), in the buttock (transverse gluteal) fold center.

Tips & References: Between the biceps femoris and the semitendinosus.

☆ About 14 cun superior to the knee fold (popliteal crease).

☆ Search for the deep depression that can be felt when moving superiorly along the thigh posterior midline.

Note: ....

~ Yinmen ~ UB 37

Location: 6 cun distal to the inferior buttock (transverse gluteal) fold, between the biceps femoris and the semitendinosus.

Tips & References: On the line connecting UB 36 and UB 40.

Note: ....

~ Fuxi ~ UB 38

Location: When the knee is slightly flexed, 1 cun proximal to the knee fold (popliteal crease), medial to the biceps femoris.

Tips & References: 1 cun proximal to UB 39.

Note: ....

~ Weiyang ~ UB 39

Location: When the knee is slightly flexed, in the knee joint, medial to the biceps femoris.

Tips & References: On the knee fold (popliteal crease) lateral side.

☆ About 1 cun lateral to UB 40.

Basic Feature: TW(SJ) lower 'He' sea pt..

Note: ....

~ Weizhong ~ UB 40

Location: When the knee is slightly flexed, in the knee joint, midway between the semitendinosus and the biceps femoris.

Tips & References: In the knee fold (popliteal crease) center.

Basic Feature: 'He' sea, earth pt.. Lower and upper back command pt..

Note: ....

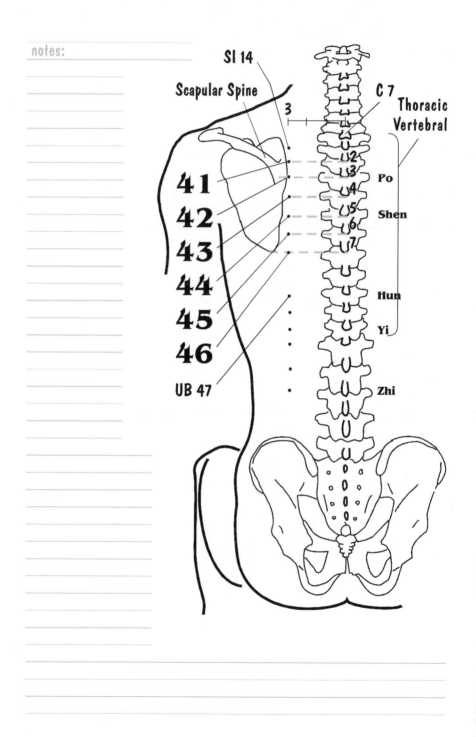

notes:

SI 14

Scapular Spine

3

C 7

Thoracic
Vertebral

41

42

43

44

45

46

UB 47

Po

Shen

Hun

Yi

Zhi

Description:

~ Fufen ~ UB 41

Location: 3 cun lateral to T2 spinous process inferior edge.
Tips & References: Vertically superior to the scapular spine medial end*.
☆   T2 spinous process is inferior to the most extended (T1) spinous process on the neck base.
☆   Vertically inferior to SI 14**. Level with UB 12.
Basic Feature: Interaction with SI.
Note: ....

~ Pohu ~ UB 42

Location: 3 cun lateral to T3 spinous process inferior edge.
Tips & References: Medial to the scapular spine medial end*.
☆   Level with UB 13 and GV(Du) 12***.
Basic Feature: "Po Gate" (Lu spiritual aspect: corporeal soul).
Note: ....

~ Gaohuangshu ~ UB 43

Location: 3 cun lateral to T4 spinous process inferior edge.
Tips & References: Vertically inferior to the scapular spine medial end*.
☆   Level with UB 14.
Note: ....

~ Shentang ~ UB 44

Location: 3 cun lateral to T5 spinous process inferior edge.
Tips & References: Vertically inferior to the scapular spine medial end*.
☆   Level with UB 15 and GV(Du) 11***.
Basic Feature: "Shen Gate" (H spiritual aspect: mind).
Note: ....

~ Yixi ~ UB 45

Location: 3 cun lateral to T6 spinous process inferior edge.
Tips & References: Vertically inferior to the scapular spine medial end*.
☆   Level with UB 16 and GV(Du) 10***.
Note: ....

~ Geguan ~ UB 46

Location: 3 cun lateral to T7 spinous process inferior edge.
Tips & References: Vertically inferior to the scapular spine medial end*.
☆   Level with the scapular inferior edge.
☆   Level with UB 17 and GV(Du) 9***.
Note: ....

* When the arm lies straight alongside the body (adduction).
** See p. 72.   *** See p. 166.

Urinary Bladder Meridian

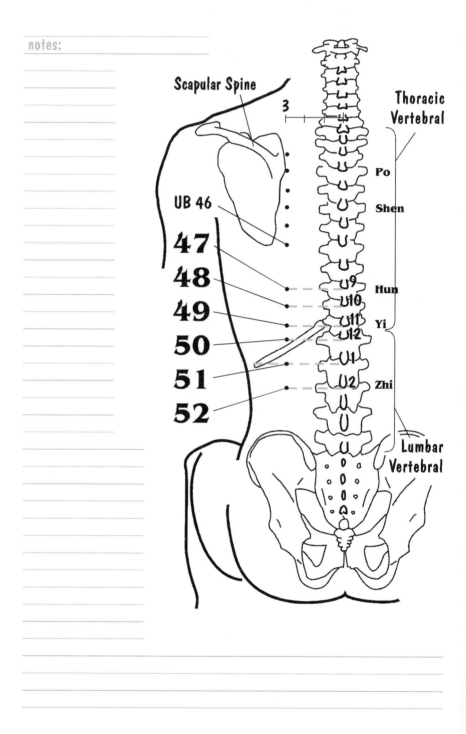

notes:

Description:

~ Hunmen ~ UB 47

Location: 3 cun lateral to T9 spinous process inferior edge.
Tips & References: Vertically inferior to the scapular spine medial end*.
☆ Level with UB 18 and GV(Du) 8**.
Basic Feature: "Hun Gate" (LIV spiritual aspect: ethereal soul).
Note: ....

~ Yanggang ~ UB 48

Location: 3 cun lateral to T10 spinous process inferior edge.
Tips & References: Vertically inferior to the scapular spine medial end*.
☆ Level with UB 19 and GV(Du) 7**.
Note: ....

~ Yishe ~ UB 49

Location: 3 cun lateral to T11 spinous process inferior edge.
Tips & References: Vertically inferior to the scapular spine medial end*.
☆ Level with UB 20 and GV(Du) 6**.
Basic Feature: "Yi Gate" (Sp spiritual aspect: mental house).
Note: ....

~ Weicang ~ UB 50

Location: 3 cun lateral to T12 spinous process inferior edge.
Tips & References: Vertically inferior to the scapular spine medial end*.
☆ Level with UB 21.
Note: ....

~ Huangmen ~ UB 51

Location: 3 cun lateral to L1 spinous process inferior edge.
Tips & References: Vertically inferior to the scapular spine medial end*.
☆ Level with the 12th rib free end.
☆ Level with UB 22 and GV(Du) 5***.
Note: ....

~ Zhishi ~ UB 52

Location: 3 cun lateral to L2 spinous process inferior edge.
Tips & References: Vertically inferior to the scapular spine medial end*.
☆ Level with UB 23 and GV(Du) 4***.
Basic Feature: "Zhi Gate" (K spiritual aspect: will power room).
Note: ....

* When the arm lies straight alongside the body (adduction).
** See p. 166.   *** See p. 164.

Urinary Bladder Meridian

notes:

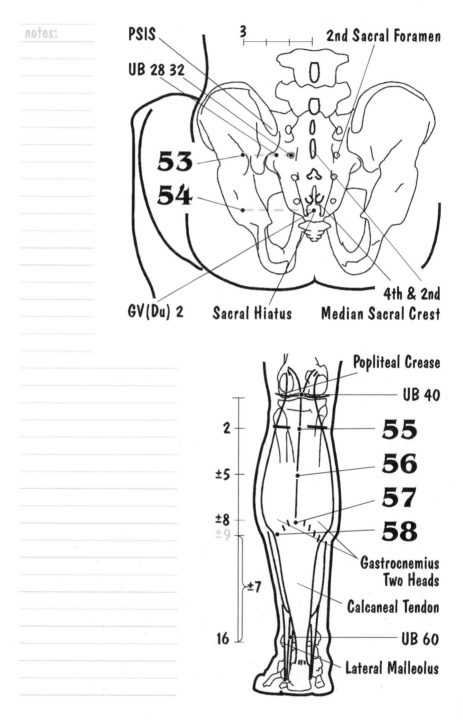

PSIS

UB 28 32

3

2nd Sacral Foramen

53

54

GV(Du) 2　　Sacral Hiatus

4th & 2nd
Median Sacral Crest

Popliteal Crease

UB 40

2

55

±5

56

57

±8
±9

58

Gastrocnemius
Two Heads

±7

Calcaneal Tendon

16

UB 60

Lateral Malleolus

Description:

~ Baohuang ~ UB 53

Location: Level with the 2nd sacral foramen, 3 cun lateral to the back midline.

Tips & References: Level with UB 28 and UB 32.

☆ Twice of the distance from the back midline to the PSIS medial border.

☆ Search for the point's depression that can be felt when moving laterally from S2 (the 2nd median sacral crest) inferior part.

Note: ....

~ Zhibian ~ UB 54

Location: Level with the sacral hiatus center, 3 cun lateral to the back midline.

Tips & References: Level with GV(Du) 2.

☆ Search for the point's depression that can be felt when moving laterally from S4 (the 4th median sacral crest) inferior border.

Note: ....

~ Heyang ~ UB 55

Location: Between the two heads of the gastrocnemius, 2 cun distal to knee fold (popliteal crease).

Tips & References: Vertically inferior to UB 40.

☆ On the line connecting UB 40 and UB 57.

Note: ....

~ Chengjin ~ UB 56

Location: Midway between UB 55 and UB 57.

Tips & References: In the center of the gastrocnemius mass.

☆ Vertically inferior to UB 40.

☆ About 5 cun inferior to the knee fold (popliteal crease) and UB 40.

Note: ....

~ Chengshan ~ UB 57

Location: At the connecting point of the Achilles (calcaneal) tendon with the two heads of the gastrocnemius.

Tips & References: About 8 cun inferior to knee fold (popliteal crease) and UB 40 (about level with the midpoint between the knee fold and the lateral malleolus).

☆ A distal stretch of the foot (plantar flexion) emphasizes this connection point.

Note: ....

~ Feiyang ~ UB 58

Location: 1 cun lateral and 1 cun distal to UB 57.

Tips & References: On the border between the gastrocnemius lateral head and the Achilles (calcaneal) tendon.

☆ On the gastrocnemius.

☆ About 7 cun superior to UB 60.

Basic Feature: 'Luo' connecting pt.. Many sources indicate interaction with K.

Note: ....

~ Points on Foot Taiyang ~
Urinary Bladder Meridian

notes:

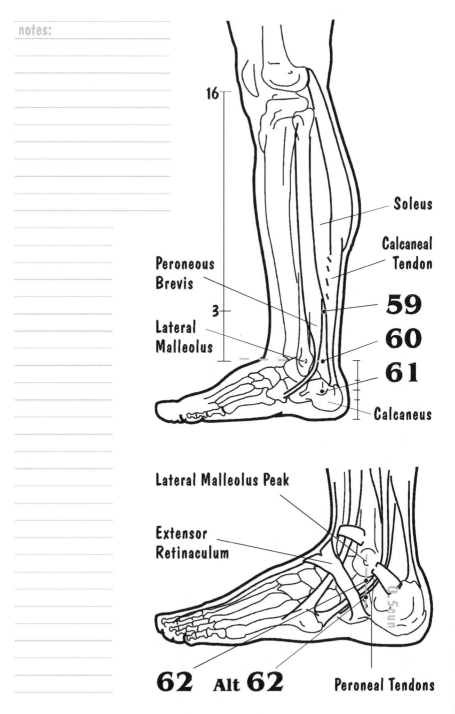

16

Soleus

Calcaneal
Tendon

Peroneous
Brevis

3

Lateral
Malleolus

59

60

61

Calcaneus

Lateral Malleolus Peak

Extensor
Retinaculum

62 Alt 62

Peroneal Tendons

Description:

~ Fuyang ~ UB 59

Location: Anterior to the Achilles (calcaneal) tendon, level with 3 cun proximal to the lateral malleolus peak.
Tips & References: 3 cun proximal to UB 60.
☆ Posterior to the proneal tendons (proneous brevis).
☆ Search for the gap end that can be felt when moving superiorly from the lateral malleolus posterior border.
Basic Feature: Yangqiao (Ya-H) 'Xi' accumulation pt..
Note: ....

~ Kunlun ~ UB 60

Location: In the depression, between the lateral malleolus and the Achilles (calcaneal) tendon, level with the lateral malleolus peak.
Tips & References: Search for the point when the foot is at a right angle to the leg.
Basic Feature: 'Jing' river, fire pt..
Note: ....

~ Pucan ~ UB 61

Location: In the depression, vertically inferior to UB 60, on the borderline between the sole skin and pigmented skin.
Tips & References: 1.5 cun inferior to UB 60.
☆ Level with the midpoint between the lateral malleolus peak and the foot sole.
☆ Search for the vertical slit end (superior to a bulge) on the calcaneus that can be felt when moving inferiorly from UB 60.
Basic Feature: Interaction with Yangqiao (Ya-H).
Note: ....

~ Shenmai ~ UB 62

Location: Inferior to the lateral malleolus, vertically inferior to the malleolus peak.
Tips & References: Between the peroneal tendons and the malleolus.
☆ Easier to identify the proneal tendons when stretching the foot distally (plantar flexion).
Alternative Location: Vertically inferior to the lateral malleolus peak, posterior (and inferior) to the peroneal tendons.
☆ About 0.5 cun inferior to lateral malleolus inferior border.
Basic Feature: Yangqiao (Ya-H) opening and starting pt.. GV (Du) coupled pt..
Note: ....

Urinary Bladder Meridian

notes:

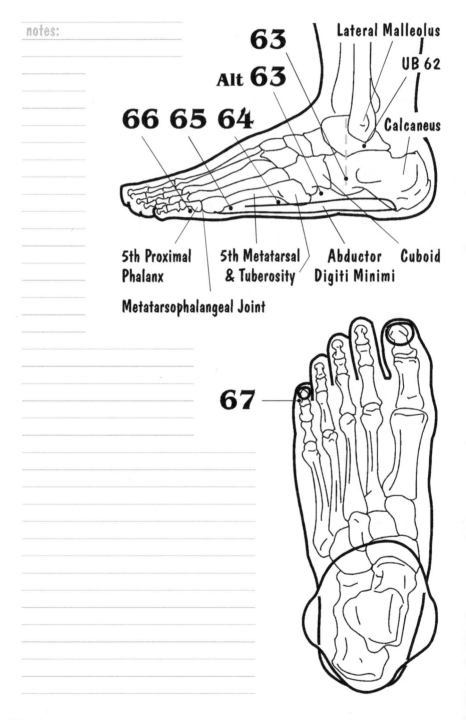

63

Lateral Malleolus

Alt 63

UB 62

66 65 64

Calcaneus

5th Proximal Phalanx

5th Metatarsal & Tuberosity

Abductor Digiti Minimi

Cuboid

Metatarsophalangeal Joint

67

Description:

~ Jinmen ~ UB 63

Location: In the depression, vertically inferior to the lateral malleolus anterior border, posterior to the cuboid.

Tips & References: About 1 cun inferior (and anterior) to UB 62.

☆ On the calcaneus, anterior to a bone bulge (peroneal trochlea of calcaneus).

Alternative Location: Inferior to the cuboid bone, vertically inferior to the cuboid center.

☆ Posterior to the 5th metatarsal bone base tuberosity. This tuberosity is the most extended structure on the foot lateral aspect.

☆ Search for the depression inferior to a vertical bone gap.

Basic Feature: 'Xi' accumulation pt.. Yangwei (Ya-L) starting point.

Note: ....

~ Jinggu ~ UB 64

Location: Anterior to the 5th metatarsal bone base tuberosity, inferior to the bone neck.

Tips & References: The 5th metatarsal tuberosity is the most extended structure on the foot lateral aspect.

☆ On the borderline between the sole skin and pigmented skin.

Basic Feature: 'Yuan' source pt..

Note: ....

~ Shugu ~ UB 65

Location: Posterior to the 5th metatarsal bone head, inferior to the bone neck.

Tips & References: Posterior to the 5th metatarsophalangeal joint.

☆ On the borderline between the sole skin and pigmented skin.

☆ Search for the first depression that can be felt when moving anteriorly along the 5th metatarsal inferior border.

Basic Feature: 'Shu' stream, wood, sedation pt..

Note: ....

~ Zutonggu ~ UB 66

Location: In the depression, anterior to the 5th proximal phalanx bone base, inferior to the bone neck.

Tips & References: Anterior to the 5th metatarsophalangeal joint.

☆ On the borderline between the sole skin and pigmented skin.

Basic Feature: 'Ying' spring, water, horary pt..

Note: ....

~ Zhiyin ~ UB 67

Location: 0.1 cun proximal to the little toenail lateral corner.

Tips & References: Proximal to the nail base.

Basic Feature: 'Jing' well, metal, tonification pt..

Note: ....

Kidney Meridian

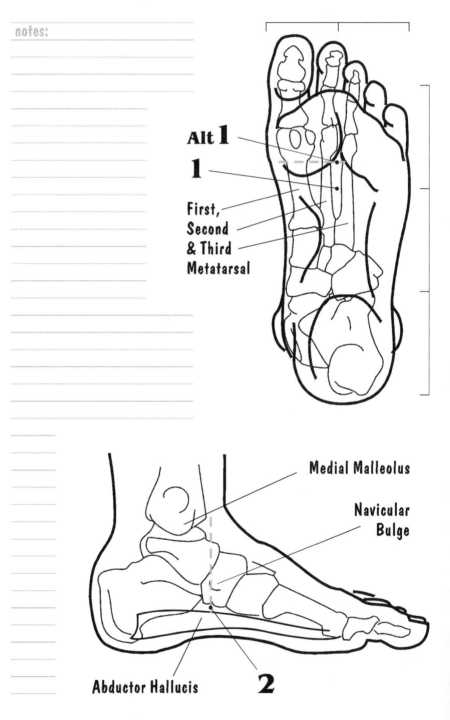

notes:

Alt 1

1

First,
Second
& Third
Metatarsal

Medial Malleolus

Navicular
Bulge

Abductor Hallucis   2

Description:

~ Yongquan ~ K 1

Location: On the sole, between the 2nd and 3rd metatarsal bones, 1/3 of the distance between the base of the 2nd toe and the heel.

Tips & References: Approximately midway of the foot width.

☆ Search for the deep depression that is formed when the foot is stretched distally (plantar flexion).

Alternative Location: On the sole, between the 2nd and 3rd metatarsal bones, level with the 1st metatarsal bone head proximal border.

☆ Search for the first deep depression that can be felt when moving proximally along the foot midline.

Basic Feature: 'Jing' well, wood, sedation pt..

Note: ....

~ Rangu ~ K 2

Location: On the navicular bone inferior border, vertically inferior to the navicular bulge.

Tips & References: Vertically inferior to the medial malleolus anterior border.

☆ On the borderline between the sole skin and pigmented skin.

☆ Inferior to a vertical slit on the navicular bone.

Basic Feature: 'Ying' spring, fire pt..

Note: ....

Kidney Meridian

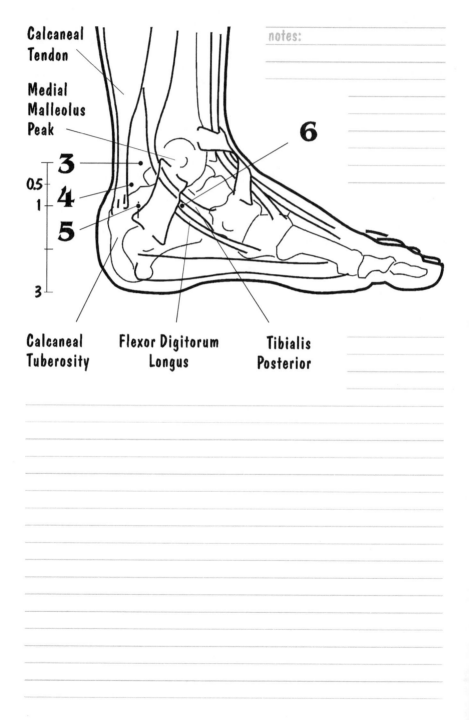

notes:

Calcaneal Tendon

Medial Malleolus Peak

3

0.5
1

4

5

6

3

Calcaneal Tuberosity

Flexor Digitorum Longus

Tibialis Posterior

Description:

~ Taixi ~ K 3

Location: In the gap, midway between the medial malleolus peak and the Achilles (calcaneal) tendon posterior border, level with the malleolus peak.

Tips & References: Between the Achilles tendon and the medial malleolus.

☆   Search for the point when the foot is loose and at a right angle to the leg.

Basic Feature: 'Shu' stream, earth pt.. 'Yuan' source pt..

Note: ....

~ Dazhong ~ K 4

Location: Anterior to the Achilles (calcaneal) tendon, superior to the calcaneus.

Tips & References: Level with 0.5 cun inferior to the medial malleolus peak.

☆   Anterior and superior to the Achilles tendon attachment.

☆   Search for the deep depression that can be felt when moving posterior-inferiorly from the medial malleolus.

Basic Feature: 'Luo' connecting pt..

Note: ....

~ Shuiquan ~ K 5

Location: Vertically inferior to the gap between the medial malleolus and the Achilles (calcaneal) tendon, level with 1 cun inferior to the medial malleolus peak.

Tips & References: 1 cun inferior to K 3.

☆   When the foot is loose and at a right angle to the leg, level with K 6.

☆   Search for the point at the superior end of a vertical slit on the calcaneus that can be felt when moving inferiorly from K 3, after passing a small bulge on the calcaneus bone.

Basic Feature: 'Xi' accumulation pt..

Note: ....

~ Zhaohai ~ K 6

Location: In the depression, 1 cun inferior to the medial malleolus peak.

Tips & References: 0.4 cun inferior to the medial malleolus inferior border.

☆   Between the flexor digitorum longus tendon (which is sometimes hard to locate) and the tibialis posterior tendon.

☆   Easier to identify the tendons when flexing the foot upward (dorsi flexion) and inwards (inversion).

☆   When the foot is loose and at a right angle to the leg, level with K 5.

☆   Search for the point in a vertical gap that lies deeply behind the two tendons.

Basic Feature: Yinqiao (Yi-H) starting and opening pt.. CV(Ren) coupled pt..

Note: ....

Kidney Meridian

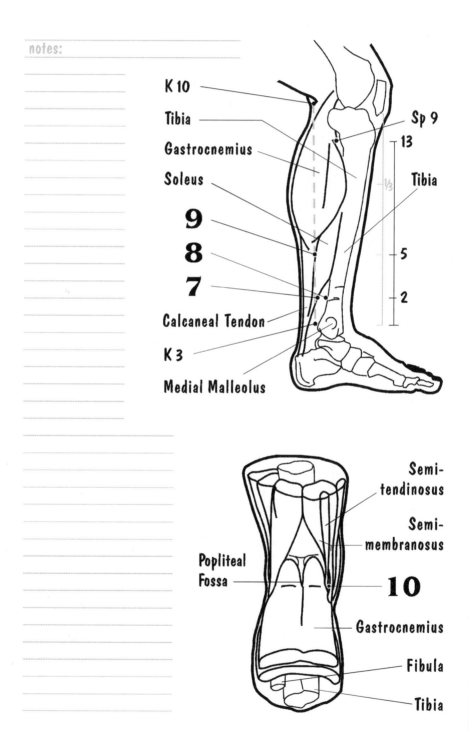

notes:

K 10

Tibia

Gastrocnemius

Soleus

9

8

7

Calcaneal Tendon

K 3

Medial Malleolus

Sp 9

13

Tibia

5

2

1/3

Semi-tendinosus

Semi-membranosus

Popliteal Fossa

10

Gastrocnemius

Fibula

Tibia

Description:

~ Fuliu ~ K 7

Location: Anterior to the Achilles (calcaneal) tendon, level with 2 cun superior to the medial malleolus peak.

Tips & References: 2 cun superior to K 3

☆　0.5 cun posterior to the tibia and K 8.

☆　Search for a horizontal slit that can be felt when moving superiorly along the tibia's posterior border.

Basic Feature: 'Jing' river, metal, tonification pt..

Note: ....

~ Jiaoxin ~ K 8

Location: Posterior to the tibia, level with 2 cun superior to the medial malleolus peak.

Tips & References: 0.5 cun anterior to the Achilles (calcaneal) tendon and K 7.

☆　Search for the point posterior to the connecting tissue, slightly behind the area where the bone is clearly felt.

☆　Search for a horizontal gap that can be felt when moving superiorly along the tibia's posterior border.

Basic Feature: Yinqiao (Yi-H) 'Xi' accumulation pt..

Note: ....

~ Zhubin ~ K 9

Location: Between the soleus and the gastrocnemius, level with 5 cun superior to the medial malleolus peak.

Tips & References: On a line connecting K 3 and K 10.

☆　Level with the gastrocnemius mass inferior border.

☆　1 cun posterior to the tibia.

☆　Level with 1/3 of the distance between the medial malleolus peak to the knee joint and the popliteal crease.

Basic Feature: Yinwei (Yi-L) starting and 'Xi' accumulation pt..

Note: ....

~ Yingu ~ K 10

Location: When the knee is bent, in the knee joint, between the semitendinosus and the semimembranosus tendons.

Tips & References: On the medial side of the popliteal fossa.

☆　Level with UB 40*.

Basic Feature: 'He' sea, water, horary pt..

Note: ....

* See p. 88.

notes:

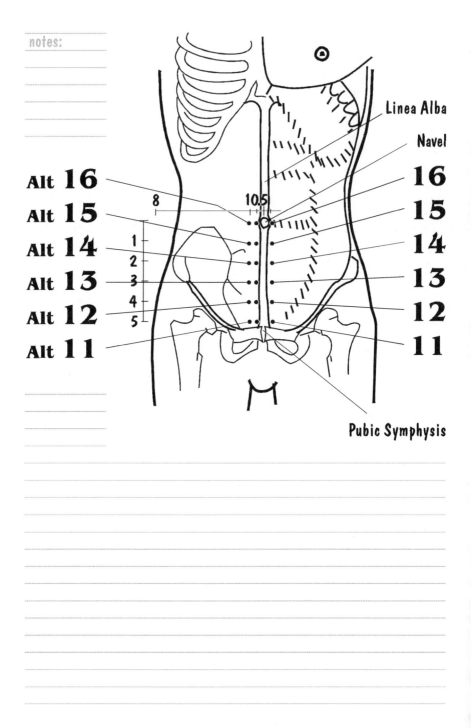

Linea Alba

Navel

Alt **16**

Alt **15**

Alt **14**

Alt **13**

Alt **12**

Alt **11**

8   10.5

1
2
3
4
5

16

15

14

13

12

11

Pubic Symphysis

Description:

~ Henggu ~ K 11

Location: 0.5 cun lateral to the front midline, level with the pubic symphysis superior border*.
Tips & References: Level with CV(Ren) 2**.
Alternative Location: 1 cun lateral to the pubic symphysis superior midpoint.
Basic Feature: Interaction with Chong (Pen.).
Note: ....

~ Dahe ~ K 12

Location: .5 cun lateral to the front midline*, level with 4 cun inferior to the navel.
Tips & References: Level with CV(Ren) 3**.
Alternative Location: 1 cun lateral to the front midline, level with 4 cun inferior to the navel.
Basic Feature: Interaction with Chong (Pen.).
Note: ....

~ Qixue ~ K 13

Location: .5 cun lateral to the front midline*, level with 3 cun inferior to the navel.
Tips & References: Level with CV(Ren) 4**.
Alternative Location: 1 cun lateral to the front midline, level with 3 cun inferior to the navel.
Basic Feature: Interaction with Chong (Pen.).
Note: ....

~ Siman ~ K 14

Location: .5 cun lateral to the front midline*, level with 2 cun inferior to the navel.
Tips & References: Level with CV(Ren) 5**.
Alternative Location: 1 cun lateral to the front midline, level with 2 cun inferior to the navel.
Basic Feature: Interaction with Chong (Pen.).
Note: ....

~ Zhongzhu ~ K 15

Location: .5 cun lateral to the front midline*, level with 1 cun inferior to the navel.
Tips & References: Level with CV(Ren) 7**.
Alternative Location: 1 cun lateral to the front midline, level with 1 cun inferior to the navel.
Basic Feature: Interaction with Chong (Pen.).
Note: ....

~ Huangshu ~ K 16

Location: 0.5 cun lateral to navel center*.
Tips & References: Level with CV(Ren) 8**.
Alternative Location: 1 cun lateral to navel center.
Basic Feature: Interaction with Chong (Pen.).
Note: ....

* On the lateral border of the front midline (linea alba) groove.   ** See p. 156.

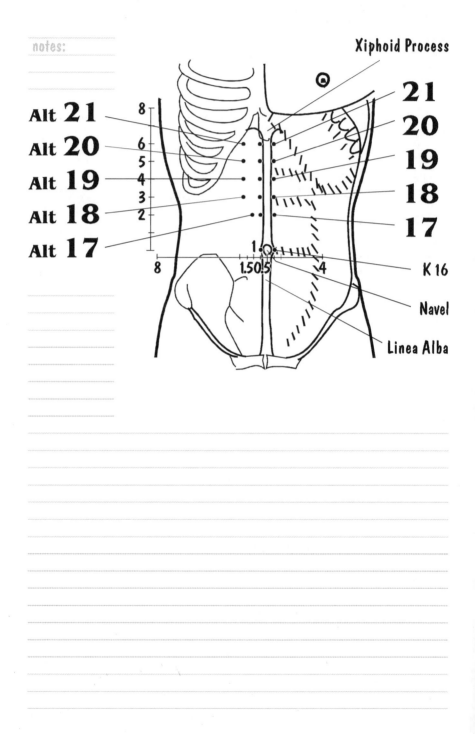

notes:

Xiphoid Process

Alt **21**
Alt **20**
Alt **19**
Alt **18**
Alt **17**

21
20
19
18
17

K 16

Navel

Linea Alba

Description:

~ Shangqu ~ K 17

Location: 0.5 cun lateral to the front midline*, level with 2 cun superior to the navel.
Tips & References: Level with CV(Ren) 10**.
Alternative Location: 1 cun lateral to the midline, level with 2 cun superior to the navel.
Basic Feature: Interaction with Chong (Pen.).
Note: ....

~ Shiguan ~ K 18

Location: 0.5 cun lateral to the front midline*, level with 3 cun superior to the navel.
Tips & References: Level with CV(Ren) 11**.
Alternative Location: 1.5 cun lateral to the midline, level with 3 cun superior to the navel.
Basic Feature: Interaction with Chong (Pen.).
Note: ....

~ Yindu ~ K 19

Location: 0.5 cun lateral to the front midline*, level with 4 cun superior to the navel.
Tips & References: Level with CV(Ren) 12**.
Alternative Location: 1.5 cun lateral to the midline, level with 4 cun superior to the navel.
Basic Feature: Interaction with Chong (Pen.).
Note: ....

~ Futonggu ~ K 20

Location: 0.5 cun lateral to the front midline*, level with 5 cun superior to the navel.
Tips & References: Level with CV(Ren) 13**.
Alternative Location: 1.5 cun lateral to the midline, level with 5 cun superior to the navel.
Basic Feature: Interaction with Chong (Pen.).
Note: ....

~ Youmen ~ K 21

Location: 0.5 cun lateral to the front midline*, level with 6 cun superior to the navel.
Tips & References: Level with CV(Ren) 14**.
☆   Normally, level with the xiphoid process inferior border.
Alternative Location: 1.5 cun lateral to the midline, level with 6 cun superior to the navel.
Basic Feature: Interaction with Chong (Pen.).
Note: ....

* On the lateral border of the front midline (linea alba) groove.
** See p. 158.

notes:

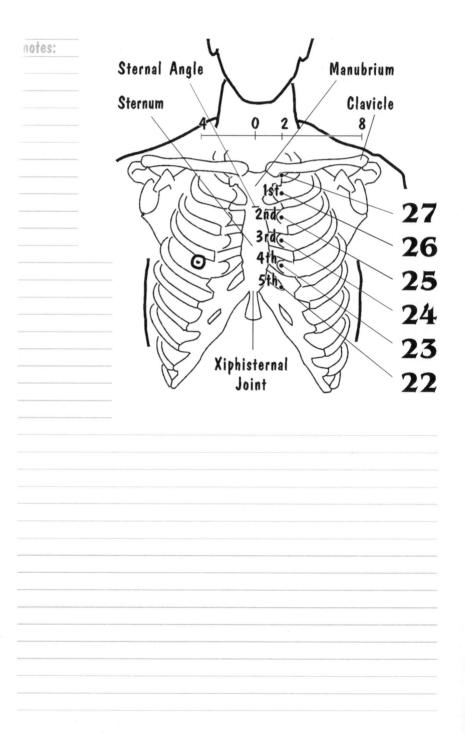

Sternal Angle

Manubrium

Sternum

Clavicle

4 0 2 8

1st.

2nd.

3rd.

4th.

5th.

27

26

25

24

23

Xiphisternal
Joint

22

Description:

~ Bulang ~ K 22

Location: In the 5th intercostal, 2 cun lateral to the front midline.

Tips & References: In the depression formed by the costal cartilage that connects the ribs to the sternum.

☆ Search for the 5th intercostal level with the xiphisternal joint.

Note: ....

~ Shenfeng ~ K 23

Location: In the 4th intercostal, 2 cun lateral to the front midline.

Tips & References: Lateral to the sternum.

☆ Male's nipple is level with the 4th intercostal, and the point is midway between the nipple to the front midline.

Note: ....

~ Lingxu ~ K 24

Location: In the 3rd intercostal, 2 cun lateral to the front midline.

Tips & References: Lateral to the sternum.

☆ The 3rd intercostal is the second space inferior to the 2nd rib which is level with the sternal angle.

Note: ....

~ Shencang ~ K 25

Location: In the 2nd intercostal, 2 cun lateral to the front midline.

Tips & References: Lateral to the sternum.

☆ The 2nd intercostal is inferior to the 2nd rib which is level with the sternal angle.

Note: ....

~ Yuzhong ~ K 26

Location: In the 1st intercostal, 2 cun lateral to the front midline.

Tips & References: Lateral to the manubrium.

☆ The 1st intercostal is superior to the 2nd rib which is level with the sternal angle.

Note: ....

~ Shufu ~ K 27

Location: Inferior to the clavicle, 2 cun lateral to the front midline.

Tips & References: Search for the second and deeper depression that can be felt when moving laterally from the manubrium superior part.

Note: ....

Pericardium Meridian

notes:

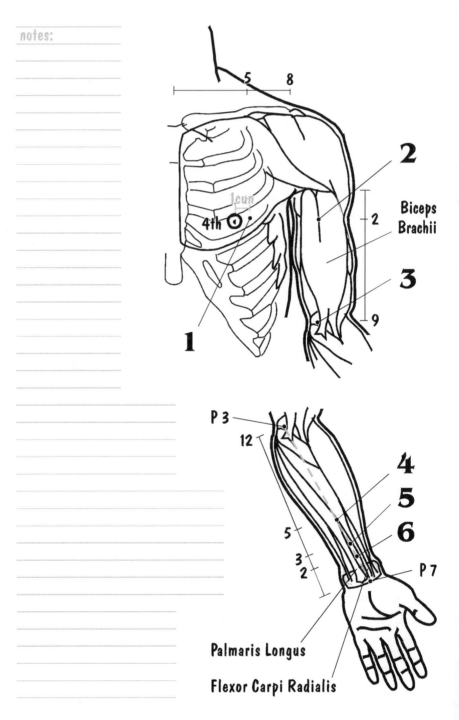

2

Biceps
Brachii

3

1

4th

1cun

5   8

P 3
12

4
5
6

5

3
2

P 7

Palmaris Longus

Flexor Carpi Radialis

Description:

~ Tianchi ~ P 1

Location: 1 cun lateral to the nipple center.
Tips & References: In the 4th intercostal
☆ 5 cun lateral to the front midline
Basic Feature: Window to the Sky. Many sources indicate interaction with GB and some indicate also interaction with Liv and TW(SJ).
Note: ....

~ Tianquan ~ P 2

Location: Between the two heads of the biceps brachii, 2 cun distal to the armpit crease (axillary fold) anterior end.
Tips & References: Easier to identify the point when arm is loose.
Note: ....

~ Quze ~ P 3

Location: When the elbow is slightly flexed, in the elbow (cubital) joint, ulnar to the biceps brachii tendon.
Tips & References: In the elbow fold.
Basic Feature: 'He' sea, water pt..
Note: ....

~ Ximen ~ P 4

Location: 5 cun proximal to the carpal groove (wrist crease), between the palmeris longus and the flexor carpi radialis tendons.
Tips & References: On the line connecting P 3 with P 7.
☆ Easier to identify the two tendons when tightening the hand.
Basic Feature: 'Xi' accumulation pt..
Note: ....

~ Jianshi ~ P 5

Location: 3 cun proximal to the carpal groove (wrist crease), between the palmeris longus and the flexor carpi radialis tendons.
Tips & References: On the line connecting P 3 with P 7.
☆ Easier to identify the two tendons when tightening the hand.
Basic Feature: 'Jing' river, metal pt.. A few sources indicate interaction with arm's three Yin meridians (Lu, H, P).
Note: ....

~ Neiguan ~ P 6

Location: 2 cun proximal to the carpal groove (wrist crease), between the palmeris longus and the flexor carpi radialis tendons.
Tips & References: On the line connecting P 3 with P 7.
☆ Easier to identify the two tendons when tightening the hand.
Basic Feature: 'Luo' connecting pt.. Yinwei (Yi-L) opening pt.. Chong (Pen.) coupled pt..
Note: ....

Pericardium Meridian

notes:

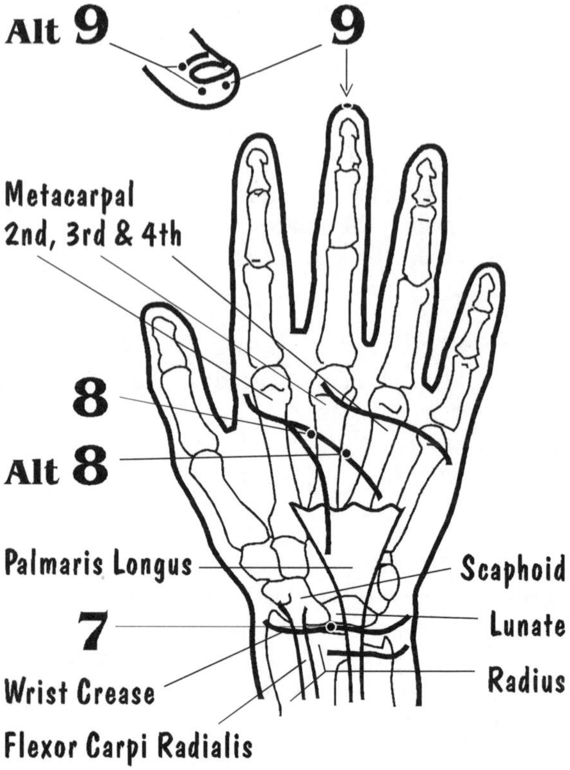

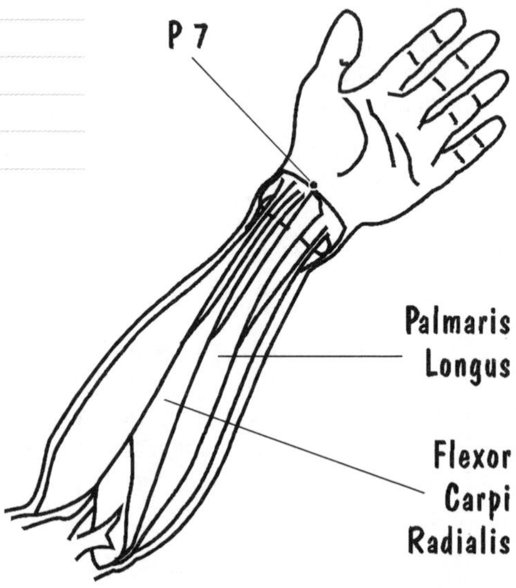

Alt **9**   **9**

Metacarpal
2nd, 3rd & 4th

8

Alt **8**

Palmaris Longus ——————— Scaphoid

7 ———————————— Lunate

Wrist Crease ———————— Radius

Flexor Carpi Radialis

P 7

Palmaris
Longus

Flexor
Carpi
Radialis

Description:

~ Daling ~ P 7

Location: In the wrist (carpal) joint, between the palmaris longus and the flexor carpi radialis tendons.

Tips & References: Easier to identify the two tendons when tightening the hand.

☆ Normally, in the carpal (wrist) crease which is not necessarily the biggest fold.

☆ At the meeting point of three bones: scaphoid, lunate and radius.

☆ Easier to identify the carpal joint when manipulating the hand.

Basic Feature: 'Shu' stream, earth, sedation pt.. 'Yuan' source pt..

Note: ....

~ Laogong ~ P 8

Location: In the depression, between the 2nd and 3rd metacarpal bones, proximal to the bone heads.

Tips & References: Radial to the 3rd metacarpal.

☆ On the palm transverse crease.

☆ When fisting the hand, where the tip of the middle (3rd) finger rests.

Alternative Location: In the depression, at the palm center.

☆ Between the 3rd and 4th metacarpal bones.

☆ Ulnar to the 3rd metacarpal.

☆ When fisting the hand, where the tip of the ring (4th) finger rests.

Basic Feature: 'Ying' spring, fire, horary pt..

Note: ....

~ Zhongchong ~ P 9

Location: At the middle (3rd) finger tip.

Alternative Location: On the radial aspect of the middle finger tip, chive leaf distal to the nail corner.

Alternative Location: 0.1 cun proximal to the middle fingernail radial corner.

☆ Proximal to the nail base.

Basic Feature: 'Jing' well, wood, tonification pt..

Note: ....

Triple Warmer (Sanjiao) M.

notes:

1

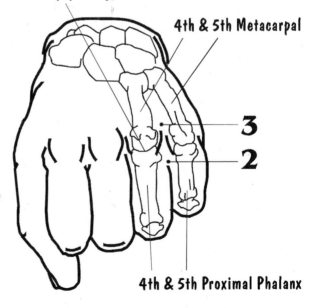

Metacarpophalangeal Joint

4th & 5th Metacarpal

3

2

4th & 5th Proximal Phalanx

Description:

~ Guanchong ~ TW(SJ) 1

Location: 0.1 cun proximal to the ulnar corner of the ring fingernail.
Tips & References: Proximal to the nail base.
Basic Feature: 'Jing' well, metal pt..
Note: ....

~ Yemen ~ TW(SJ) 2

Location: When the hand is fisted, between the ring and little fingers, distal to the 4th and 5th proximal phalanges bone bases.
Tips & References: distal to the metacarpophalangeal joint.
☆ On the borderline between the palm skin and pigmented skin.
☆ Midpoint between the web margin and the metacarpophalangeal joint line.
☆ Search for the point at the end of a soft tissue that can be felt when moving proximally between the two fingers toward the metacarpophlangeal joint.
Basic Feature: 'Ying' spring, water pt..
Note: ....

~ Zhongzhu ~ TW(SJ) 3

Location: When the hand is fisted, between the 4th and 5th metacarpal bones, proximal to the bone heads.
Tips & References: Proximal to the metacarpophalangeal joints.
☆ About 0.4 cun proximal to the midpoint between the most protruding point on the 4th and the 5th metacarpophalangeal joints.
☆ Search for the second depression that can be felt when moving proximally from the 4th and the 5th metacarpophalangeal joints along the gap between the metacarpal bones.
Basic Feature: 'Shu' stream, wood, tonification pt..
Note: ....

Triple Warmer (Sanjiao) M.

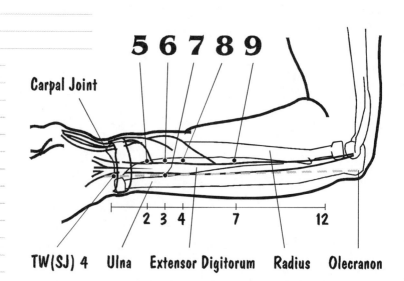

Extensor
Digiti
Minimi

4

Extensor
Digitorum

4th and
5th
Metacarpals

Alt 4

5 6 7 8 9

Carpal Joint

2 3 4   7   12

TW(SJ) 4   Ulna   Extensor Digitorum   Radius   Olecranon

Description:

~ Yangchi ~ TW(SJ) 4

Location: On the wrist (carpal) joint, ulnar to the extensor digitorum tendon.

Tips & References: Radial to the extensor digiti minimi tendon.

☆   When fisting and stretching the hand, two depressions appear (and disappear) on the wrist dorsal aspect. The point is in the ulnar one.

☆   Search for the depression in the wrist joint that can be felt when moving proximally along the gap between the 4th and 5th metacarpals.

Alternative Location: On the wrist (carpal) joint, radial to the extensor digitorum.

☆   When fisting and stretching the hand, two depressions appear (and disappear) on the wrist dorsal aspect. The point is in the radial one.

Basic Feature: 'Yuan' source pt..

Note: ....

~ Waiguan ~ TW(SJ) 5

Location: When the hand rests on the belly, 2 cun proximal to the wrist (carpal) joint, between the extensor digitorum and the radius.

Basic Feature: 'Luo' connecting pt.. Yangwei (Ya-L) opening pt.. Dai (Gir.) coupled pt.

Note: ....

~ Zhigou ~ TW(SJ) 6

Location: When the hand rests on the belly, 3 cun proximal to the wrist (carpal) joint, between the extensor digitorum and the radius.

Basic Feature: 'Jing' river, fire, horary pt..

Note: ....

~ Huizong ~ TW(SJ) 7

Location: When the hand rests on the belly, 3 cun proximal to the wrist (carpal) joint, between the extensor digitorum and the ulna.

Tips & References: 1 finger breadth (3rd finger) ulnar to TW(SJ) 6.

☆   On the line connecting TW(SJ) 4 with the olecranon peak.

Basic Feature: 'Xi' accumulation pt..

Note: ....

~ Sanyangluo ~ TW(SJ) 8

Location: When the hand rests on the belly, 4 cun proximal to the wrist (carpal) joint, radial to the extensor digitorum.

Tips & References: Ulnar to the radius.

Basic Feature: A few sources indicate interaction with the arm's three Yang meridians (LI, TW(SJ) and SI).

Note: ....

~ Sidu ~ TW(SJ) 9

Location: When the hand rests on the belly, 7 cun proximal to the wrist (carpal) joint, radial to the extensor digitorum.

Tips & References: Between the ulna and the radius.

Note: ....

Triple Warmer (Sanjiao) M.

notes:

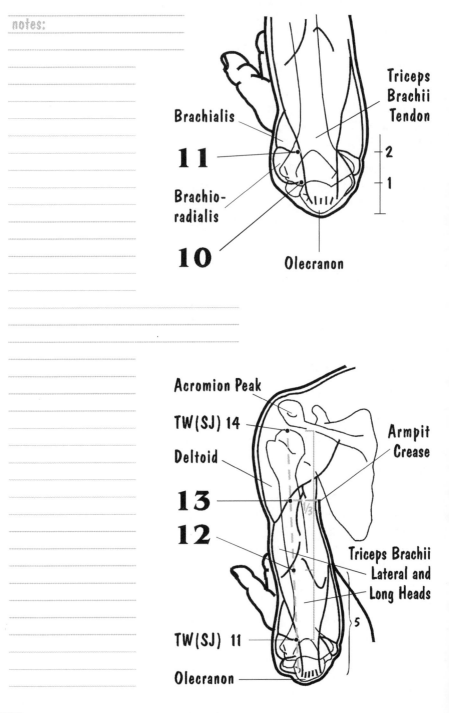

Triceps
Brachii
Tendon

Brachialis

11

2

1

Brachio-
radialis

10

Olecranon

Acromion Peak

TW(SJ) 14

Armpit
Crease

Deltoid

13

12

Triceps Brachii
Lateral and
Long Heads

5

TW(SJ) 11

Olecranon

Description:

~ Tianjing ~ TW(SJ) 10

Location: When the elbow is flexed and the palm faces the superior (supination), lateral to the triceps brachii tendon, about 1 cun proximal to the olecranon peak.

Tips & References: Search for the first depression that can be felt when moving superiorly from the olecranon peak, along the triceps brachii tendon lateral border.

Basic Feature: 'He' sea, earth, sedation pt..

Note: ....

~ Qinglengyuan ~ TW(SJ) 11

Location: When the elbow is flexed and the palm faces the superior (supination), lateral to the triceps brachii tendon, 2 cun proximal to the olecranon peak.

Tips & References: 1 cun proximal to TW(SJ) 10.

☆ In the depression, between the brachialis and brachioradialis muscles.

☆ Search for the second depression that can be felt when moving superiorly from the olecranon peak, along the triceps brachii tendon lateral border.

Note: ....

~ Xiaoluo ~ TW(SJ) 12

Location: On the line connecting the olecranon with TW(SJ) 14, midway between TW(SJ) 11 and TW(SJ) 13.

Tips & References: About 1/3 of the distance between TW(SJ) 11 to TW(SJ) 14.

☆ About 5 cun proximal to the olecranon or 7 cun inferior to the acromion peak.

☆ Between the triceps brachii long head and the triceps brachii lateral head.

☆ The point's depression is distinct when turning the arm inwards (pronation).

☆ Search for the gap end that can be felt when moving proximally from the olecranon toward the acromion.

Note: ....

~ Naohui ~ TW(SJ) 13

Location: On the line connecting the olecranon with TW(SJ) 14, posterior (and inferior) to the deltoid.

Tips & References: About 2/3 of the distance between TW(SJ) 11 to TW(SJ) 14.

☆ 3 cun distal to TW(SJ) 14.

☆ Normally, level with the armpit crease (axillary fold) posterior end.

Basic Feature: Some sources indicate interaction with Yangwei (Ya-L) and a few indicate also interaction with LI.

Note: ....

Triple Warmer (Sanjiao) M.

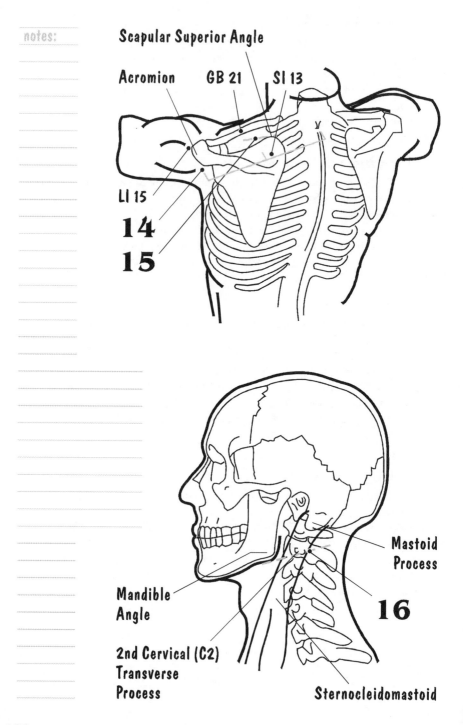

Scapular Superior Angle

Acromion   GB 21   SI 13

LI 15

14

15

Mastoid
Process

Mandible
Angle

16

2nd Cervical (C2)
Transverse
Process

Sternocleidomastoid

Description:

~ Jianliao ~ TW(SJ) 14

Location: In the depression, about 0.3 cun Inferior (and distal) to the acromion posterior-lateral corner.

Tips & References: When the arm is horizontal and loose (abduction), two curved depressions appear on the shoulder. The point is in the posterior one beneath the bone.

☆   When the arm is lifted, about 1 cun posterior to LI 15*.

☆   Search for the second small depression that can be felt when moving distally from the acromion posterior corner.

Note: ....

~ Tianliao ~ TW(SJ) 15

Location: In the depression, midway between GB 21** and SI 13***.

Tips & References: Level with the scapular superior angle.

☆   Vertically superior to the midpoint between the acromion lateral end and back midline.

Basic Feature: Interaction with GB and Yangwei (Ya-L).

Note: ....

~ Tianyou ~ TW(SJ) 16

Location: Posterior to the sternocleidomastoid, level with the mandible angle.

Tips & References: On the line continuing posteriorly the jaw inferior border.

☆   The sternocleidomastoid muscle of one side is more distinct when the head is turned to the other side and resisting a pressure applied (e.g. on the chin) from the first side.

☆   Lateral to C2 transverse process.

☆   Search for C2 transverse process that can be felt as a first process when moving inferiorly, about 1.5 cun, from the mastoid along the sternocleidomastoid posterior border.

Basic Feature: Window to the Sky.

Note: ....

* See p. 28.
** See p. 136.
*** See p. 72.

Triple Warmer (Sanjiao) M.

notes:

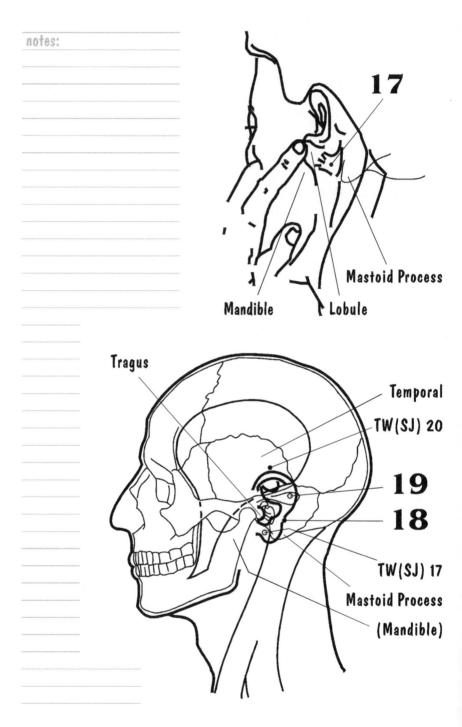

17

Mastoid Process

Mandible   Lobule

Tragus

Temporal

TW(SJ) 20

19
18

TW(SJ) 17

Mastoid Process

(Mandible)

Description:

~ Yifeng ~ TW(SJ) 17

Location: Behind the ear lobe (lobule), in the depression between the mandible and the mastoid process.
Basic Feature: Interaction with GB. Expels wind.
Note: ....

~ Qimai ~ TW(SJ) 18

Location: Behind the ear (helix), in the small horizontal slit on the temporal bone, 1/3 of the curved distance when following the arch around the ear and starting from TW(SJ) 17 to TW(SJ) 20.
Tips & References: Level with the tragus inferior end and GB 2*.
☆ Search for the point's depression that can be felt when moving superiorly from the mastoid process center.
Note: ....

~ Luxi ~ TW(SJ) 19

Location: Behind the ear (helix), on the temporal bone, 2/3 of the curved distance when following the arch around the ear and starting from TW(SJ) 17 to TW(SJ) 20.
Tips & References: Search for the point's depression beyond a bone bulge that can be felt when moving superiorly (and slightly posterior) from TW(SJ) 18.
Note: ....

* See p. 128.

Triple Warmer (Sanjiao) M.

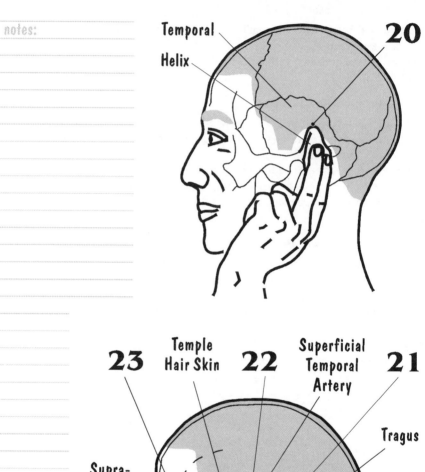

Temporal

Helix

20

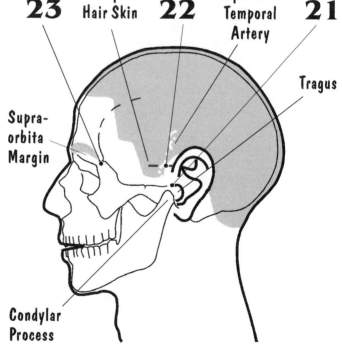

23 Temple Hair Skin **22** Superficial Temporal Artery **21**

Tragus

Supra-orbita Margin

Condylar Process

Description:

~ Jiaosun ~ TW(SJ) 20

Location: In the depression on the temporal bone, superior to the ear auricle superior tip (auricle apex).

Tips & References: Within the hair line.

☆ Easier to identify the auricle superior tip when the ear (helix) is folded anteriorly (with the ear posterior border resting on the ear anterior border).

Basic Feature: Interaction with GB and some sources indicate also interaction with SI.

Note: ....

~ Ermen ~ TW(SJ) 21

Location: When the mouth is slightly open, between the ear cartilage and the condylar process, level with the tragus superior edge.

Tips & References: Posterior and vertically superior to the condylar process.

Note: ....

~ Erheliao ~ TW(SJ) 22

Location: On the posterior temple hairline, level with the auricle root superior border.

Tips & References: posterior to or on the superficial temporal artery (search for the sensation of pulse).

☆ About 0.5 cun anterior to the ear.

☆ The hairline is the borderline between a regular skin tissue and the oilier hair-skin tissue. This borderline can be felt when running the fingernail on the skin.

Basic Feature: Interaction with SI and GB.

Note: ....

~ Sizhukong ~ TW(SJ) 23

Location: In the depression on the eyebrow lateral end.

Tips & References: On the supraorbital margin.

☆ Search for the point in a vertical slit that can be felt when moving laterally along the eyebrow.

Note: ....

Gall Bladder Meridian

notes:

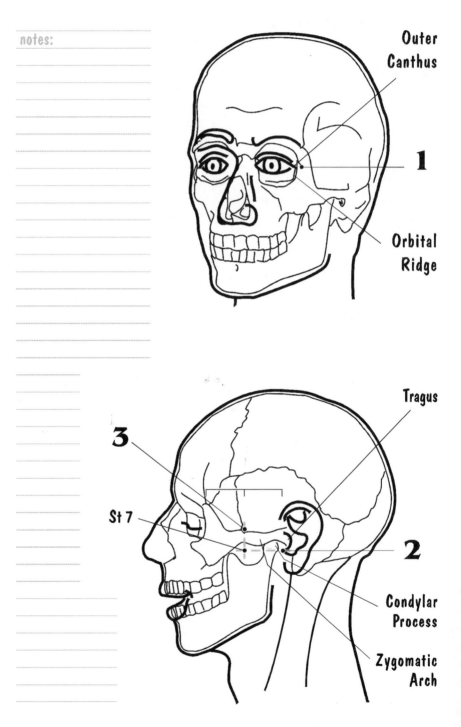

Outer Canthus

1

Orbital Ridge

Tragus

3

St 7

2

Condylar Process

Zygomatic Arch

~ Acupoint Location Guide ~

Description:

~ Tongziliao ~ GB 1

Location: In the depression, on the lateral aspect of the orbital ridge, level with the outer canthus.

Tips & References: About 0.5 cun lateral to the eye outer canthus.

☆   Level with a horizontal slit on the lateral orbital ridge center.

☆   Search for the flat area lateral to the orbital ridge; the point is located at its anterior limit.

Basic Feature: Interaction with TW(SJ) and SI.

Note: ....

~ Tinghui ~ GB 2

Location: When the mouth is wide open, between the ear cartilage and the condylar process, level with the tragus inferior notch

Tips & References: Search for the condylar process inferior border with the mouth closed, then, in the depression that appears when opening the mouth widely.

Note: ....

~ Shangguan ~ GB 3

Location: Superior to the vertical slit on the zygomatic arch superior border.

Tips & References: Vertically superior to zygomatic arch center and St 7.

☆   Search for the vertical slit that can be felt when moving anteriorly along the zygomatic arch superior border.

Basic Feature: Interaction with St and TW(SJ).

Note: ....

~ Points on Foot Shaoyang ~
Gall Bladder Meridian

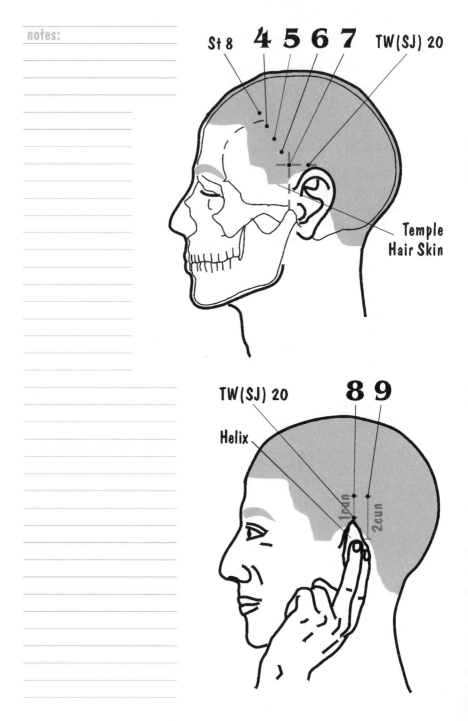

St 8 **4 5 6 7** TW(SJ) 20

Temple
Hair Skin

TW(SJ) 20 **8 9**

Helix

1cun

2cun

Description:

~ Hanyan ~ GB 4

Location: 1/4 of the distance between St 8* and GB 7.
Tips & References: Easier to feel the point while chewing.
Basic Feature: Interaction with St and TW(SJ) and some sources indicate also interaction with LI.
Note: ....

~ Xuanlu ~ GB 5

Location: Midway between St 8* and GB 7.
Basic Feature: Some sources indicate interaction with LI, St and TW(SJ).
Note: ....

~ Xuanli ~ GB 6

Location: 3/4 of the distance between St 8* and GB 7.
Basic Feature: Interaction with LI, St and TW(SJ).
Note: ....

~ Qubin ~ GB 7

Location: Vertically superior to the ear cartilage anterior border, level with auricle apex superior border.
Tips & References: About 1 finger breadth anterior to TW(SJ) 20**.
Basic Feature: Interaction with UB.
Note: ....

~ Shuaigu ~ GB 8

Location: On the head temple aspect, in the depression, 1 cun superior to the ear auricle edge (apex).
Tips & References: Easier to identify the auricle superior edge when the ear (helix) is folded anteriorly (with the ear posterior border resting on the ear anterior border).
☆   1 cun superior to TW(SJ) 20**.
☆   1.5 cun superior to the hairline***.
Basic Feature: Interaction with UB.
Note: ....

~ Tianchong ~ GB 9

Location: In the depression, vertically superior to the ear root posterior border, 2 cun superior the hairline***.
Tips & References: About 0.5 cun posterior to GB 8.
☆   GB 8, 9, 10, 11 and 12 are on one curved line.
Basic Feature: Interaction with UB.
Note: ....

* See p. 34.   ** See p. 126.
*** The hairline is the borderline between a regular skin tissue and the oilier hair-skin tissue. This borderline can be felt when running the fingernail on the skin.

Gall Bladder Meridian

notes:

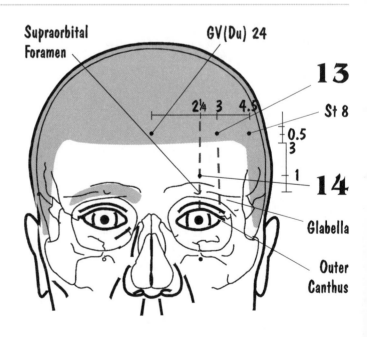

GB 9

10

11

Occipit
Protuberance

Alt 11

Mastoid
Process

Sterno-
cleidomastoid

12

Supraorbital
Foramen

GV(Du) 24

13

2¼ 3   4.5

St 8

0.5
3

1

14

Glabella

Outer
Canthus

Description:

~ Fubai ~ GB 10

Location: In the depression, 1/3 of the curved distance when following the arch around the ear starting from GB 9 to GB 12.

Tips & References: Posterior and superior to the mastoid process.

Basic Feature: Interaction with UB.

Note: ....

~ Touqiaoyin ~ GB 11

Location: In the depression, 2/3 of the curved distance when following the arch around the ear starting from GB 9 to GB12.

Tips & References: Posterior to the mastoid process.

☆ Level with the occipit protuberance inferior border.

☆ Search for the first deep depression that can be felt when moving posterior-superiorly along the mastoid posterior border.

Alternative Location: In the depression on the temporal bone, about 3/4 of the curved distance when following the arch around the ear from GB 9 to GB12.

☆ Posterior to the mastoid process.

Basic Feature: Interaction with UB and some sources indicate also interaction with TW(SJ) and SI.

Note: ....

~ Wangu ~ GB 12

Location: In the depression, posterior and inferior to the mastoid process.

Tips & References: <u>On</u> the sternocleidomastoid.

☆ Easier to identify the point's depression when bending the head forward.

Basic Feature: Many sources indicate interaction with UB.

Note: ....

~ Benshen ~ GB 13

Location: 0.5 cun superior to the forehead hairline*, 3 cun lateral to the head midline.

Tips & References: 1/3 of the distance between St 8*** to GV(Du) 24**.

☆ Vertically superior to the eye outer canthus.

Basic Feature: Interaction with Yangwei (Ya-L).

Note: ....

~ Yangbai ~ GB 14

Location: In the depression, 1 cun superior to the supraorbital foramen.

Tips & References: The supraorbital foramen is under the eyebrow center.

☆ Vertically superior to the pupil center when looking straight ahead.

☆ 2.25 cun lateral to the front midline.

☆ Level with 1/3 of the distance between the glabella to the forehead hairline*.

Basic Feature: Interaction with Yangwei (Ya-L) and some sources indicate also interaction with LI, St and TW(SJ).

Note: ....

* The limit between the hair-skin tissue and the regular skin tissue can be felt by moving the fingernail upward on the forehead (hair-skin tissue is oilier).
** See p. 170.   *** See p. 34.

Gall Bladder Meridian

notes:

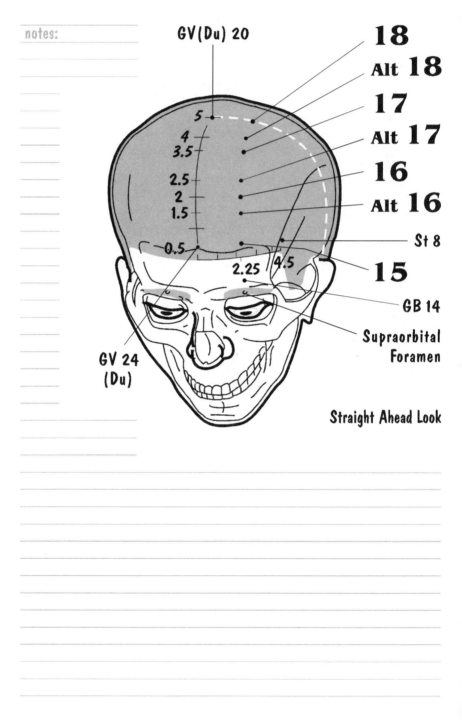

GV(Du) 20

18

Alt **18**

17

Alt **17**

16

Alt **16**

St 8

15

GB 14

Supraorbital Foramen

5

4
3.5

2.5
2
1.5

0.5

2.25   4.5

GV 24
(Du)

Straight Ahead Look

Description:

~ Toulinqi ~ GB 15

Location: 2.25 cun lateral to the head midline, 0.5 cun superior to the forehead hairline*.

Tips & References: Midway between GV(Du) 24*** and St 8****.

☆ Vertically superior to the pupil's center when looking straight ahead**.

Basic Feature: Interaction with UB and Yangwei (Ya-L).

Note: ....

~ Muchuang ~ GB 16

Location: 2.25 cun lateral to the head midline, 2 cun superior to the forehead hairline*.

Tips & References: 1.5 cun posterior to GB 15.

☆ Vertically posterior to the pupil's center when looking straight ahead**.

Alternative Location: 2.25 cun lateral to the front midline, 1.5 cun superior to the forehead hairline.

Basic Feature: Interaction with Yangwei (Ya-L).

Note: ....

~ Zhengying ~ GB 17

Location: 2.25 cun lateral to the head midline, 3.5 cun posterior to the forehead hairline*.

Tips & References: 3 cun posterior to GB 15, 1.5 cun posterior to GB 16.

☆ Vertically posterior to the pupil's center when looking straight ahead**.

Alternative Location: 2.25 cun lateral to the front midline, 2.5 cun posterior to the forehead hairline.

Basic Feature: Interaction with Yangwei (Ya-L).

Note: ....

~ Chengling ~ GB 18

Location: 2.25 cun lateral to the head midline, 5 cun posterior to the forehead hairline*.

Tips & References: 4.5 cun posterior to GB 15, 1.5 cun posterior to GB 17.

☆ Vertically posterior to the pupil's center when looking straight ahead**.

☆ Vertically superior to the ear auricle posterior border.

☆ Level with GV(Du) 20***.

☆ On the line connecting GB 15 and GB 20.

Alternative Location: 2.25 cun lateral to the head midline, 4 cun posterior to the forehead hairline.

Basic Feature: Interaction with Yangwei (Ya-L).

Note: ....

* The hairline is the borderline between a regular skin tissue and the oilier hair-skin tissue. This borderline can be felt when running the fingernail on the skin.

** Vertically superior to the supraorbital foramen that can be felt under the eyebrow center, and also vertically superior to GB14.

*** See p. 170.　　****See p. 34.

Gall Bladder Meridian

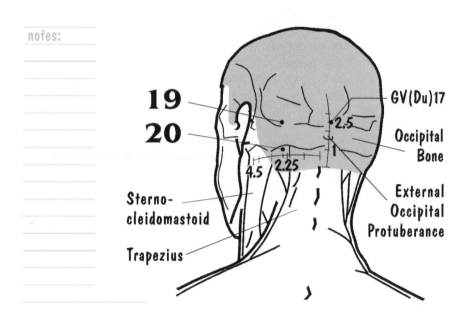

19
20

GV(Du)17

2.5

Occipital
Bone

2.25

4.5

Sterno-
cleidomastoid

External
Occipital
Protuberance

Trapezius

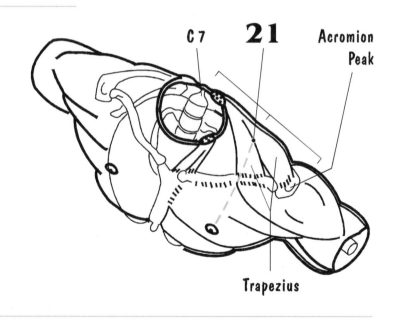

C 7   **21**   Acromion
Peak

Trapezius

Description:

~ Naokong ~ GB 19

Location: 2.25 cun lateral to the head midline, level with the external occipital protuberance superior border.

Tips & References: Vertically superior to the midpoint between the mastoid process and the neck midline

☆   1.5 cun superior to GB 20.

☆   Level with 2.5 cun superior to the neck hairline*.

☆   Level with GV(Du) 17**.

Basic Feature: Interaction with Yangwei (Ya-L).

Note: ....

~ Fengchi ~ GB 20

Location: Inferior to the occipital bone, in the depression between the sternocleidomastoid and the trapezius.

Tips & References: 2.25 cun lateral to the back midline.

☆   Midway between the mastoid process and the neck midline.

☆   Level with 1 cun superior to the neck hairline*.

☆   Level with GV(Du) 16**.

☆   Easier to identify the depression when bending the head backward.

Basic Feature: Interaction with Yangwei (Ya-L), Yangqiao (Ya-H) and some sources indicate also interaction with TW(SJ).

Note: ....

~ Jianjing ~ GB 21

Location: In the trapezius split, midway between C7 spinous process and the acromion peak.

Tips & References: C7 spinous process is the first spinous process that can be felt when moving inferiorly along the neck midline (when the head is anteriorly dropped it disappears).

☆   At the shoulder highest point.

☆   On the superior part of the shoulder but with an anterior aspect.

☆   Vertically superior to the nipple.

☆   Search for the point depression that can be felt when moving medially from the acromion along the shoulder. Note, the point is not necessarily in the deepest depression.

Basic Feature: Many sources indicate interaction with TW(SJ), Yangwei (Ya-L) and some indicate also interaction with St.

Note: ....

---

* The hairline is the borderline between a regular skin tissue and the oilier hair-skin tissue. This borderline can be felt when running the fingernail, upwards, on the skin.

** See p. 168.

Gall Bladder Meridian

notes:

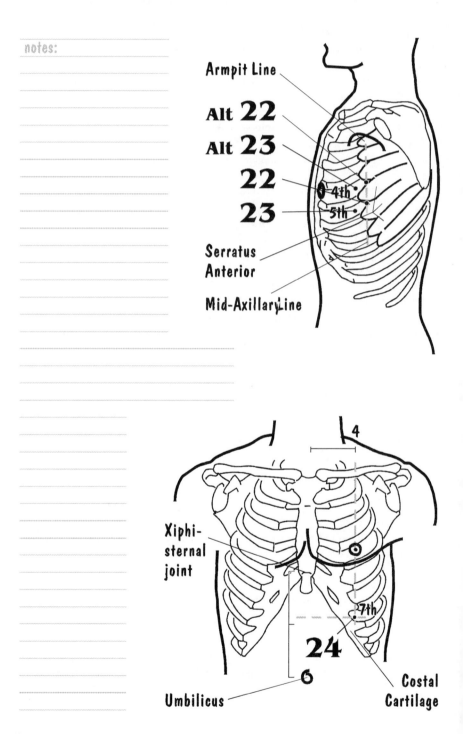

Armpit Line

Alt **22**

Alt **23**

22

23

4th

5th

Serratus
Anterior

Mid-Axillary Line

4

Xiphi-
sternal
joint

7th

24

6

Umbilicus

Costal
Cartilage

Description:

~ Yuanye ~ GB 22

Location: When the arm is raised (abduction), in the 5th intercostal, on the mid-axillary line.

Tips & References: Anterior to the serratus anterior heads.

☆ Vertically inferior to the armpit center.

☆ Search for the 5th intercostal space lateral to the xiphisternal joint.

Alternative Location: In the 4th intercostal, on the mid-axillary line.

☆ Anterior to the serratus anterior heads.

☆ Vertically inferior to the armpit center.

☆ The 4th intercostal is the first space superior to the 5th intercostal which is lateral to the xiphisternal joint.

☆ Search for the 4th intercostal space lateral to the nipple.

Note: ....

~ Zhejin ~ GB 23

Location: In the 5th intercostal, 1 cun anterior to the mid-axillary line.

Tips & References: 1 cun anterior to GB 22.

☆ 1 cun anterior to the serratus anterior heads.

☆ Search for the 5th intercostal space lateral to the xiphisternal joint.

Alternative Location: In the 4th intercostal, 1 cun anterior to the mid-axillary line.

☆ 1 cun anterior to the serratus anterior splitting heads.

☆ 1 cun anterior to Alt. GB 22.

☆ The 4th intercostal is the first space superior to the 5th intercostal which is lateral to the xiphisternal joint.

☆ Search for the 4th intercostal space lateral to the nipple.

Basic Feature: Second GB front 'Mu' collecting pt.. Some sources indicate interaction with UB.

Note: ....

~ Riyue ~ GB 24

Location: In the 7th intercostal, vertically inferior to the nipple.

Tips & References: 4 cun lateral to the front midline.

☆ On the costal cartilage lateral border.

☆ Level with 0.5 cun superior to the midpoint between umbilicus and the xiphisternal joint.

Basic Feature: GB front 'Mu' collecting pt.. Interaction with Sp and some sources indicate also interaction with Yangwei (Ya-L).

Note: ....

Gall Bladder Meridian

notes:

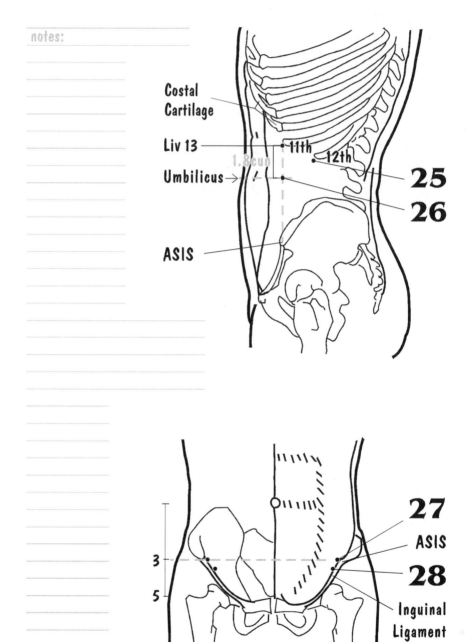

Costal
Cartilage

Liv 13

11th

1.8cun

12th

Umbilicus

25

26

ASIS

27

ASIS

28

Inguinal
Ligament

3

5

Description:

~ Jingmen ~ GB 25

Location: Anterior and inferior to the 12th rib's free end.
Tips & References: On the body lateral side, but with a posterior aspect.
Basic Feature: K front 'Mu' collecting pt..
Note: ....

~ Daimai ~ GB 26

Location: Vertically inferior to the 11th rib's free end, level with the umbilicus.
Tips & References: On the body lateral side, but with an anterior aspect.
☆ Vertically superior to the ASIS* or slightly anterior to it.
☆ 1.8 cun inferior to Liv 13**.
☆ Search for the 11th rib free end that can be felt when moving inferior-laterally along the costal cartilage medial border.
Basic Feature: Dai (Gir.) starting pt..
Note: ....

~ Wushu ~ GB 27

Location: Medial to the ASIS*.
Tips & References: On the inguinal ligament superior (and medial) border.
☆ Level with 3 cun inferior to the umbilicus.
Basic Feature: Interaction with Dai (Gir.).
Note: ....

~ Weidao ~ GB 28

Location: In the depression, superior to the inguinal ligament, about 0.5 cun medial (and inferior) to the ASIS*.
Tips & References: About 0.5 cun medial (and inferior) to GB 27.
☆ Search for the first deep depression that can be felt when moving inferior-medially from the ASIS along the inguinal ligament superior border.
Basic Feature: Interaction with Dai (Gir.).
Note: ....

* Anterior Superior Iliac Spine.
** See p. 154.

Gall Bladder Meridian

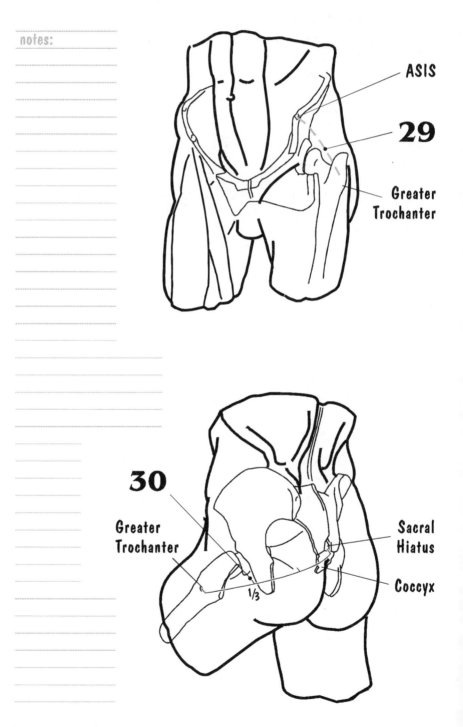

ASIS

29

Greater
Trochanter

30

Greater
Trochanter

Sacral
Hiatus

Coccyx

1/3

Description:

~ Juliao ~ GB 29

Location: In the gap, midway between the ASIS (Anterior superior Iliac Spine) and the greater trochanter peak.

Tips & References: Easier to identify the point location when lying on the side with the hip flexed.

☆   At the lateral end of the fold created when flexing the hip.

Basic Feature: Interaction with Yangqiao (Ya-H).

Note: ....

~ Huantiao ~ GB 30

Location: When the thigh is bent at a right angle (extension), 1/3 of the distance between the greater trochanter peak and the sacral hiatus.

Tips & References: The sacral hiatus depression is at the sacrum base, superior to the coccyx.

☆   Easier to locate the point when lying on the side (in a lateral recumbent position).

Basic Feature: Interaction with UB.

Note: ....

notes:

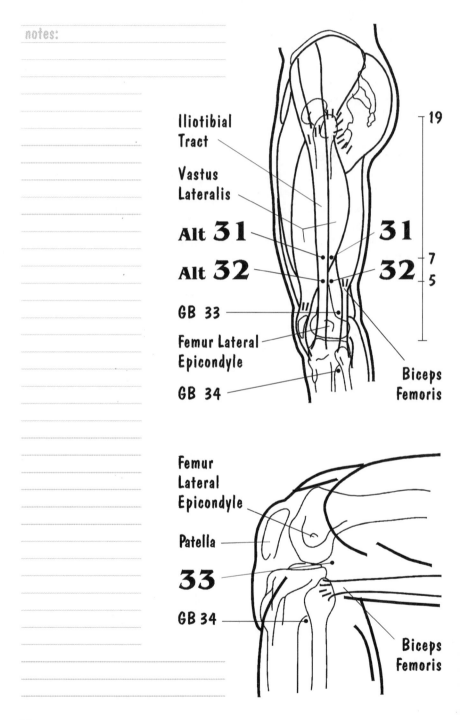

Iliotibial Tract

Vastus Lateralis

Alt 31

Alt 32

GB 33

Femur Lateral Epicondyle

GB 34

31

32

19

7
5

Biceps Femoris

Femur Lateral Epicondyle

Patella

33

GB 34

Biceps Femoris

Description:

~ Fengshi ~ GB 31

Location: On the thigh lateral midline, 7 cun superior to the knee joint and fold (popliteal crease).

Tips & References: Posterior to the iliotibial tract.

☆ When standing up with the arms alongside the body, the point is at the center of the thigh, where the middle finger tip rests (but this description may give several locations).

Alternative Location: On the thigh lateral midline, 7 cun superior to the knee fold (popliteal crease).

☆ On the iliotibial tract midline.

Note: ....

~ Zhongdu ~ GB 32

Location: On the thigh lateral midline, 5 cun superior to the knee fold (popliteal crease).

Tips & References: Between the biceps femoris muscle and the vastus lateralis muscle.

☆ Posterior to the iliotibial tract.

Alternative Location: On the thigh lateral midline, 5 cun superior to the knee fold (popliteal crease).

☆ On the iliotibial tract midline.

Note: ....

~ Xiyangguan ~ GB 33

Location: When the knee is flexed, between the femur lateral epicondyle and the biceps femoris, proximal to the knee joint.

Tips & References: Level with the patella inferior border.

☆ When the knee is straight, superior (and posterior) to the femur lateral epicondyle; about 3 cun superior to GB 34.

☆ Search at the most distal point on the border of the hollow which is formed when the knee is flexed at a right angle.

Note: ....

~ Points on Foot Shaoyang ~
Gall Bladder Meridian

notes:

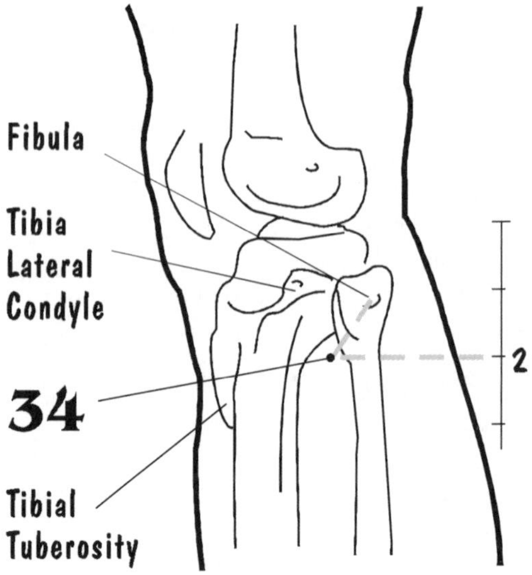
Fibula
Tibia
Lateral
Condyle
34
Tibial
Tuberosity
2

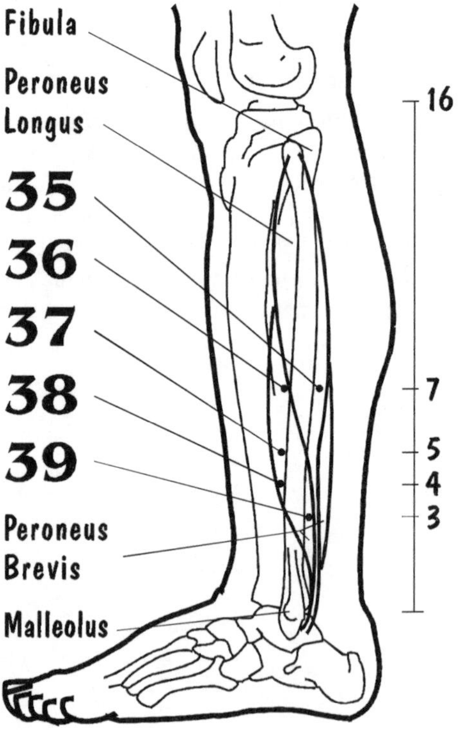
Fibula
Peroneus
Longus
35
36
37
38
39
Peroneus
Brevis
Malleolus
16
7
5
4
3

Description:

~ Yanglingquan ~ GB 34

Location: On the knee lateral aspect, anterior and distal to the fibula's head.
Tips & References: About 1 cun distal (and anterior) to the fibula head peak.
☆ Approximately, level with 2 cun inferior to the popliteal joint and crease.
☆ Search for the gap end that can be felt when moving superiorly along the anterior-lateral aspect of the lower leg.
Basic Feature: 'He' sea, earth pt.. Tendon 'Hui' gathering pt..
Note: ....

~ Yangjiao ~ GB 35

Location: 7 cun proximal to the lateral malleolus peak, posterior to the fibula.
Tips & References: Easier to identify the fibular posterior border on its inferior part.
Basic Feature: Yangwei (Ya-L) 'Xi' accumulation pt..
Note: ....

~ Waiqiu ~ GB 36

Location: 7 cun proximal to the lateral malleolus peak, anterior to the fibula.
Tips & References: Easier to identify the fibula border on its inferior part.
Basic Feature: 'Xi' accumulation pt..
Note: ....

~ Guangming ~ GB 37

Location: 5 cun proximal to the lateral malleolus peak, anterior to the fibula.
Tips & References: Easier to identify the fibular border on its inferior part.
Basic Feature: 'Luo' connecting pt..
Note: ....

~ Yangfu ~ GB 38

Location: 4 cun proximal to the lateral malleolus peak, anterior to the fibula.
Tips & References: Easier to identify the fibular border on its inferior part.
Basic Feature: 'Jing' river, fire, sedation pt..
Note: ....

~ Xuanzhong ~ GB 39

Location: 3 cun proximal to the lateral malleolus peak, posterior to the fibula.
Tips & References: Anterior to the peroneus longus.
☆ Easier to identify the peroneal tendons when stretching the foot distally (plantar flexion).
☆ Easier to identify the fibular posterior border on its inferior part.
Basic Feature: Bone marrow 'Hui' gathering pt.. Many sources indicate interaction with the leg three Yang meridians (St, UB and GB).
Note: ....

Gall Bladder Meridian

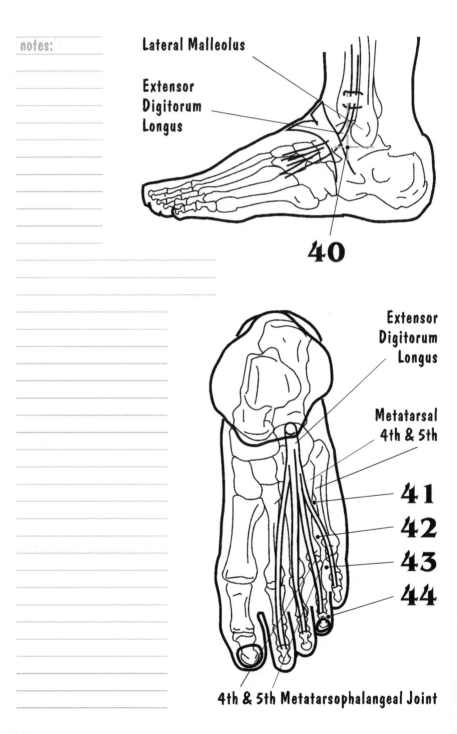

notes:

Lateral Malleolus

Extensor
Digitorum
Longus

40

Extensor
Digitorum
Longus

Metatarsal
4th & 5th

41

42

43

44

4th & 5th Metatarsophalangeal Joint

Description:

~ Qiuxu ~ GB 40

Location: When the foot is loose and at a right angle to the leg, in the depression, at the ankle joint, posterior (and inferior) to the extensor digitorum longus tendon.
Tips & References: Easier to identify the tendon when lifting (extending) the toes.
☆   Level with lateral malleolus inferior border.
☆   Vertically inferior to the lateral malleolus anterior border.
Basic Feature: 'Yuan' source pt..
Note: ....

~ Zulinqi ~ GB 41

Location: Between the 4th and 5th metatarsal bones, proximal (and lateral) to the extensor digitorum longus lateral branch.
Tips & References: Distal to the metatarsal bone bases.
☆   Easier to identify the tendon when lifting (extending) the toes.
Basic Feature: 'Shu' stream, wood, horary pt.. Dai (Gir.) opening pt.. Yangwei (Ya-L) coupled pt..
Note: ....

~ Diwuhui ~ GB 42

Location: Between the 4th and 5th metatarsal bones, distal (and medial) to the extensor digitorum longus lateral branch.
Tips & References: Proximal to the bone heads.
☆   Easier to identify the tendon when lifting (extending) the toes.
Note: ....

~ Xiaxi ~ GB 43

Location: Between the 4th and 5th toes, midway between the web margin and the metatarsophalangeal joint.
Tips & References: On the borderline between the sole skin and pigmented skin.
☆   Search for the web margin by opening a gap between the two toes.
Basic Feature: 'Ying' spring, water, tonification pt..
Note: ....

~ Zuqiaoyin ~ GB 44

Location: 0.1 cun proximal to the lateral corner of the 4th toenail.
Tips & References: Proximal to the nail base.
Basic Feature: 'Jing' well, metal pt..
Note: ....

Liver Meridian

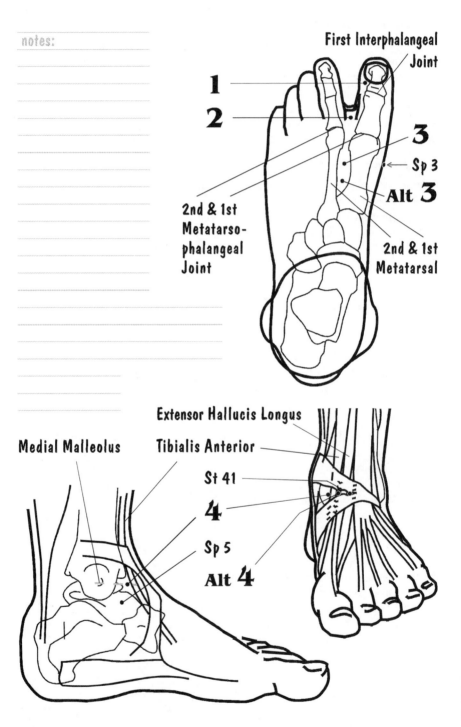

notes:

First Interphalangeal Joint

1

2

3

Sp 3

Alt 3

2nd & 1st Metatarso-phalangeal Joint

2nd & 1st Metatarsal

Extensor Hallucis Longus

Medial Malleolus

Tibialis Anterior

St 41

4

Sp 5

Alt 4

Description:

~ Dadun ~ Liv 1

Location: 0.15 cun proximal to the lateral corner of the big toenail.

Tips & References: Midway between the big toenail lateral corner and the 1st interphalangeal joint.

☆   Proximal to the nail base.

Basic Feature: 'Jing' well, wood, horary pt.. Interaction with GB.

Note: ....

~ Xingjian ~ Liv 2

Location: Between the big and 2nd toes, midway between the web margin and the metatarsophalangeal joint.

Tips & References: About 0.5 cun proximal to the web margin.

☆   On the borderline between the sole skin and pigmented skin.

☆   Search for the point while opening a gap between the two toes.

Basic Feature: 'Ying' spring, fire, sedation pt..

Note: ....

~ Taichong ~ Liv 3

Location: Between the 1st and 2nd metatarsals, proximal to the bone heads.

Tips & References: Level with Sp 3*.

☆   Search for the first deep depression that can be felt when moving proximally from the metatarsophalangeal joints along the gap beginning between the big and the second toes.

Alternative Location: Between the 1st and 2nd metatarsals, distal to the bone bases.

Basic Feature: 'Shu' stream, earth pt.. 'Yuan' source pt..

Note: ....

~ Zhongfeng ~ Liv 4

Location: At the ankle joint, medial to the tibialis anterior tendon, level with the medial malleolus peak.

Tips & References: 1 cun anterior to the medial malleolus peak.

☆   In a superior and bigger depression than Sp 5**.

☆   Midway between Sp 5** and St 41***.

☆   Search for the tendon (tibialis anterior) while bending the foot and turning it inwards (inversion).

Alternative Location: At the ankle joint, between the tibialis anterior tendon and the extensor hallucus longus tendon.

☆   Search for the tendon while bending the foot and turning it inwards (inversion).

Basic Feature: 'Jing' river, metal pt..

Note: ....

* See p. 50.   ** See p. 52.   *** See p. 48.

Liver Meridian

notes:

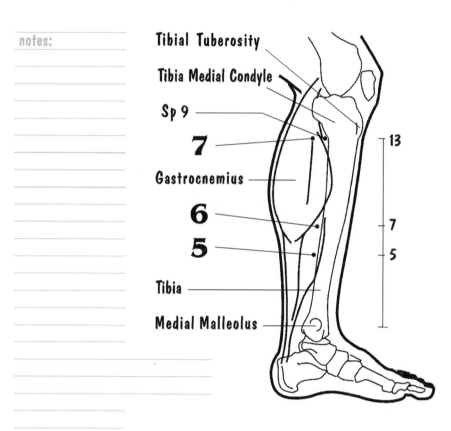

Tibial Tuberosity

Tibia Medial Condyle

Sp 9

7

Gastrocnemius

6

5

Tibia

Medial Malleolus

13

7

5

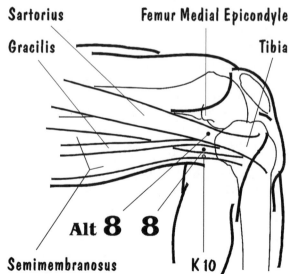

Sartorius

Gracilis

Femur Medial Epicondyle

Tibia

Alt **8** **8**

Semimembranosus

K 10

152

Description:

~ Ligou~ Liv 5

Location: On the medial aspect of the leg, 5 cun proximal to the medial malleolus peak, posterior to the tibia.

Tips & References: Search for the point behind the connecting tissue, slightly posterior to the area where the bone is clearly felt.

Basic Feature: 'Luo' connecting pt..

Note: ....

~ Zhongdu ~ Liv 6

Location: On the medial aspect of the leg, 7 cun proximal to the medial malleolus peak, posterior to the tibia.

Tips & References: Anterior to the gastrocnemius.

☆　Search for the point behind the connecting tissue, slightly posterior to the area where the bone is clearly felt.

Basic Feature: 'Xi' accumulation pt..

Note: ....

~ Xiguan ~ Liv 7

Location: On the medial aspect of the leg, 1 cun posterior to the tibial neck, level with the tibial tuberosity inferior border.

Tips & References: Posterior and inferior to the tibia medial condyle.

☆　1 cun posterior to Sp 9*.

☆　In a vertical split on the gastrocnemius.

Note: ....

~ Ququan ~ Liv 8

Location: When the knee is flexed at a right angle, on the medial aspect of the leg, between the semimembranosus tendon and the gracilis muscle, proximal to the knee joint.

Tips & References: Posterior to the femur medial epicondyle.

☆　The same level with K 10** but anterior to the semimembranosus tendon.

☆　On the line perpendicular to the knee fold (popliteal crease) medial end.

☆　Easier to identify the anatomical structure when the foot lies on the other knee and resists a pressure applied on the lifted knee medial aspect.

Alternative Location: When the knee is flexed at a right angle, midway between the semimembranosus tendon and the femur medial epicondyle, proximal to the knee joint.

☆　Search for the first deep depression that can be felt when the knee is in full flexion (the heel touches the buttock) and moving proximally from the femur medial epicondyle.

☆　Search at the most distal point on the border of the hollow which is formed when the knee is flexed at a right angle.

Basic Feature: 'He' sea, water, tonification pt..

Note: ....

* See p. 52.　　** See p. 104.

Liver Meridian

notes:

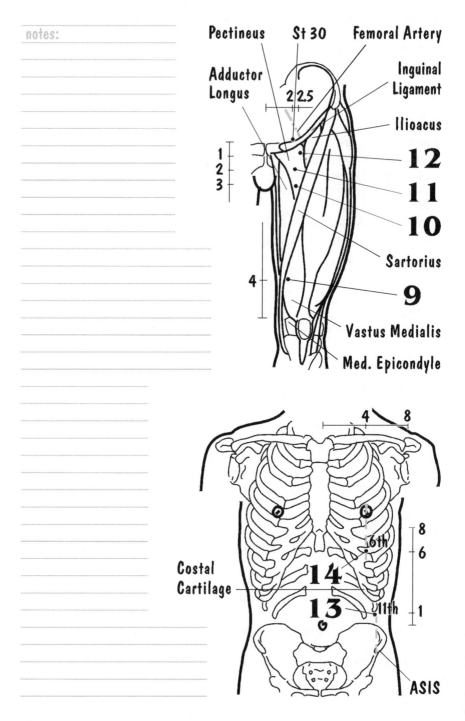

Pectineus   St 30   Femoral Artery

Adductor   Inguinal
Longus   Ligament

2 2.5

Ilioacus

12

11

10

Sartorius

9

Vastus Medialis

Med. Epicondyle

4   8

8
6

Costal
Cartilage

14

13

ASIS

Description:

~ Yinbao ~ Liv 9

Location: Level with 4 cun superior to the medial epicondyle superior border, anterior to the sartorius muscle.
Note: ....

~ Zuwuli ~ Liv 10

Location: 3 cun inferior to St 30*.
Tips & References: Anterior to the adductor longus.
☆ Medial (and superior) to the sartorius.
☆ Search for the triangle cavity distal border that can be felt when moving distally from the thigh superior part along the thigh anterior-medial midline.
Note: ....

~ Yinlian ~ Liv 11

Location: 2 cun inferior to St 30*.
Tips & References: 1 cun vertically superior to Liv 10.
Note: ....

~ Jimai ~ Liv 12

Location: In the depression, inferior to the inguinal ligament, 2.5 cun lateral to the front midline.
Tips & References: 1 cun inferior (and lateral) to St 30*.
☆ Medial to the femoral artery (search for the sensation of pulse) and vein.
Note: ....

~ Zhangmen ~ Liv 13

Location: Anterior and inferior to the 11th rib free end.
Tips & References: Normally, on the body lateral side, but with an anterior aspect.
☆ Vertically superior to the ASIS, or slightly anterior to it.
☆ Search for the 11th rib free end that can be felt when moving inferior-laterally along the costal cartilage medial border.
☆ A fast search for the 11th rib free end can start at the umbilicus, moving laterally along the body landmarks toward the costal cartilage.
Basic Feature: Sp front 'Mu' collecting pt.. 'Zang' Yin organs 'Hui' gathering pt.. Many sources indicate interaction with GB.
Note: ....

~ Qimen ~ Liv 14

Location: In the 6th intercostal, 4 cun lateral to the front midline.
Tips & References: Vertically inferior to the nipple.
☆ Level with 6 cun superior to the umbilicus.
☆ Search for the costal cartilage second and bigger depression that can be felt when moving laterally toward the 6th intercostal.
Basic Feature: Liv front 'Mu' collecting pt.. Interaction with Sp and Yinwei (Yi-L).
Note: ....

* See p. 42.

Conception Vessel

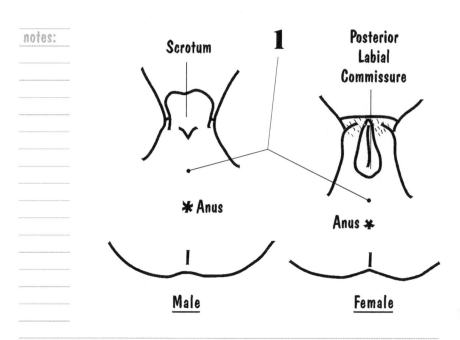

Scrotum

1

Posterior
Labial
Commissure

✳ Anus

Anus ✳

<u>Male</u>

<u>Female</u>

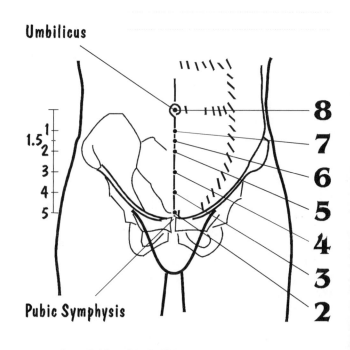

Umbilicus

8

1.5
1
2
3
4
5

7

6

5

4

Pubic Symphysis

3

2

Description:

~ Huiyin ~ CV(Ren) 1

Location:

☆ **Male:** Midway between the anus and the scrotum.

☆ **Female:** Midway between the anus and the posterior labial commissure.

Basic Feature: Chong (Pen.) opening pt.. Interaction with GV(Du).

Note: ....

~ Qugu ~ CV(Ren) 2

Location: The symphysis pubis superior border midpoint.

☆ 5 cun inferior to the umbilicus.

Basic Feature: Interaction with Liv.

Note: ....

~ Zhongji ~ CV(Ren) 3

Location: 4 cun inferior to the umbilicus center.

Basic Feature: UB front 'Mu' collecting pt.. Interaction with the leg's three Yin meridians (Sp, Liv and K) and some sources indicate also interaction with St.

Note: ....

~ Guanyuan ~ CV(Ren) 4

Location: 3 cun inferior to the umbilicus center.

Basic Feature: Sea of blood. Yuan gate. SI front 'Mu' collecting pt.. Interaction with the leg's three Yin meridians (Sp, Liv and K) and some sources indicate also interaction with St.

Note: ....

~ Shimen ~ CV(Ren) 5

Location: 2 cun inferior to the umbilicus center.

Basic Feature: TW(SJ) front 'Mu' collecting pt..

Note: ....

~ Qihai ~ CV(Ren) 6

Location: 1.5 cun inferior to the umbilicus center.

Note: ....

~ Yinjiao ~ CV(Ren) 7

Location: 1 cun inferior to the umbilicus center.

Basic Feature: Many sources indicate interaction with K and Chong (Pen.).

Note: ....

~ Shenque ~ CV(Ren) 8

Location: In the umbilicus center.

Note: ....

Conception Vessel

notes:

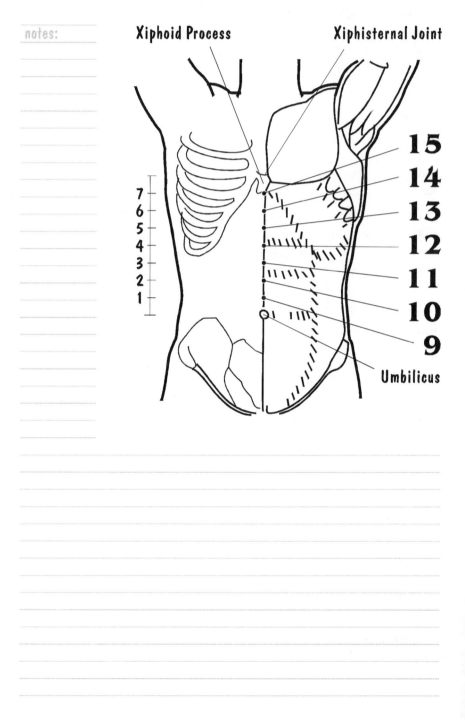

Xiphoid Process   Xiphisternal Joint

15
14
13
12
11
10
9

Umbilicus

Description:

~ Shuifen ~ CV(Ren) 9

Location: 1 cun superior to the umbilicus center.
Note: ....

~ Xiawan ~ CV(Ren) 10

Location: 2 cun superior to the umbilicus center.
Basic Feature: Interaction with Sp.
Note: ....

~ Jianli ~ CV(Ren) 11

Location: 3 cun superior to the umbilicus center.
Note: ....

~ Zhongwan ~ CV(Ren) 12

Location: 4 cun superior to the umbilicus center.
Basic Feature: 'Fu' Yang organ 'Hui' gathering pt.. St front 'Mu' collecting pt..
Interaction with St, SI and many sources indicate also interaction with TW(SJ).
Note: ....

~ Shangwan ~ CV(Ren) 13

Location: 5 cun superior to the umbilicus center.
Basic Feature: Interaction point with St and SI.
Note: ....

~ Juque ~ CV(Ren) 14

Location: 6 cun superior to the umbilicus center.
Basic Feature: H front 'Mu' collecting pt..
Note: ....

~ Jiuwei ~ CV(Ren) 15

Location: When the arms are lifted (supine position), inferior to the xiphoid process.
Tips & References: 7 cun superior to the umbilicus center.
Basic Feature: 'Xi' connecting pt..
Note: ....

Conception Vessel

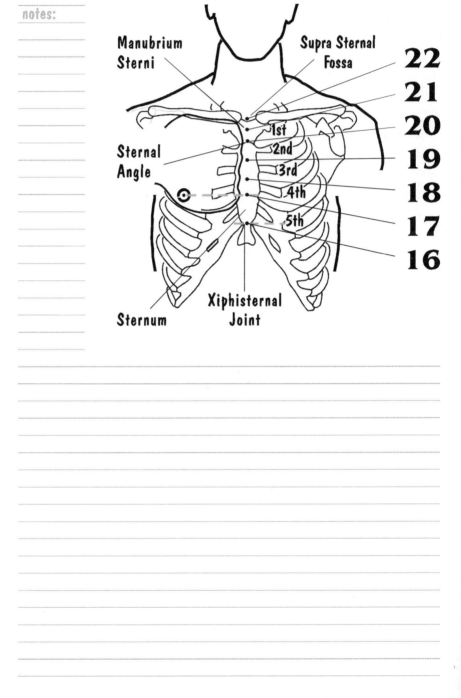

Description:

~ Zhongting ~ CV(Ren) 16

Location: On the sternum midline, level with the 5th intercostal space medial end.
Tips & References: In the xiphisternal joint center.
Note: ....

~ Danzhong ~ CV(Ren) 17

Location: On the sternum midline, level with the 4th intercostal space medial end.
Tips & References: In male, midway between the two nipples.
☆   The 5th intercostal is level with the xiphisternal joint and the 4th intercostal is the first space superior to it.
Basic Feature: Qi 'Hui' gathering pt.. P front 'Mu' collecting pt.. Sea of Qi. Interaction with SI and some sources indicate interaction with Sp, K, TW(SJ) and UB.
Note: ....

~ Yutang ~ CV(Ren) 18

Location: On the sternum midline, level with the 3rd intercostal space medial end.
Tips & References: The 3nd intercostal is the second space inferior to the 2nd rib which is level with the sternal angle.
Note: ....

~ Zigong ~ CV(Ren) 19

Location: On the sternum midline, level with the 2nd intercostal space medial end.
Tips & References: The 2nd intercostal is inferior to the 2nd rib which is level with the sternal angle.
Note: ....

~ Huagai ~ CV(Ren) 20

Location: On the sternum midline, level with the 1st intercostal space medial end.
Tips & References: The 1st intercostal is superior to the 2nd rib which is level with the sternal angle.
Note: ....

~ Xuanji ~ CV(Ren) 21

Location: In the center of the manubrium sterni.
Tips & References: Midway between CV(Ren) 20 and CV(Ren) 22.
☆   About 1 cun inferior to CV(Ren) 22 or/and 1 cun superior to CV(Ren) 20.
Note: ....

~ Tiantu ~ CV(Ren) 22

Location: In the center of the supra sternal fossa.
Tips & References: Superior to the manubrium sterni superior border.
Basic Feature: Window to the Sky. Interaction point with Yinwei (Yi-L).
Note: ....

Conception Vessel

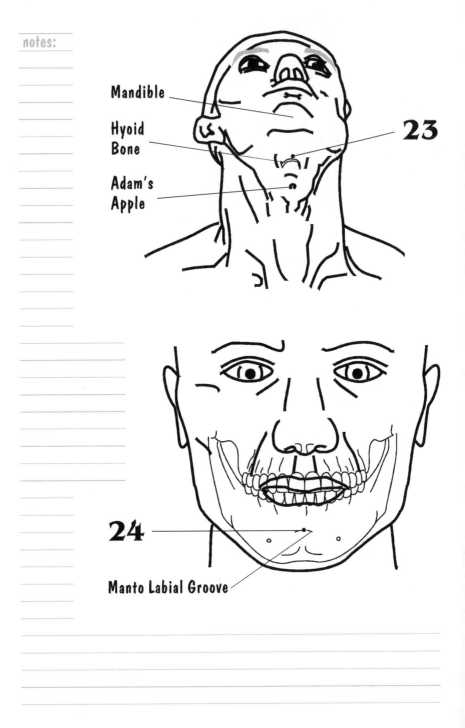

notes:

Mandible

Hyoid Bone

Adam's Apple

23

24

Manto Labial Groove

Description:

~ Lianquan ~ CV(Ren) 23

Location: In the center of the hyoid superior border.

Tips & References: Head held straight (not like in the illustration).

☆   Midway between the mandible and the Adam's apple peak.

☆   Search for the hyoid superior border that can be felt when moving posteriorly from the chin toward the throat midline.

Basic Feature: Many sources indicate interaction with Yinwei (Yi-L).

Note: ....

~ Chengjiang ~ CV(Ren) 24

Location: In the center of the manto labial groove.

☆   Puncture should be toward the superior aspect.

Basic Feature: Interaction with St and some sources indicate also interaction with LI and GV(Du).

Note: ....

Governing Vessel

notes:

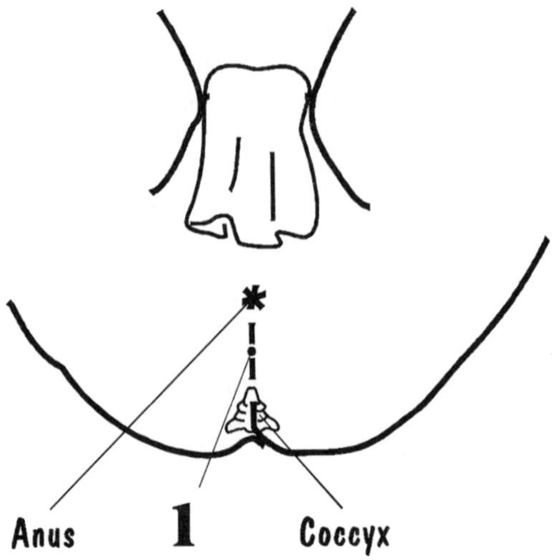

Anus   **1**   Coccyx

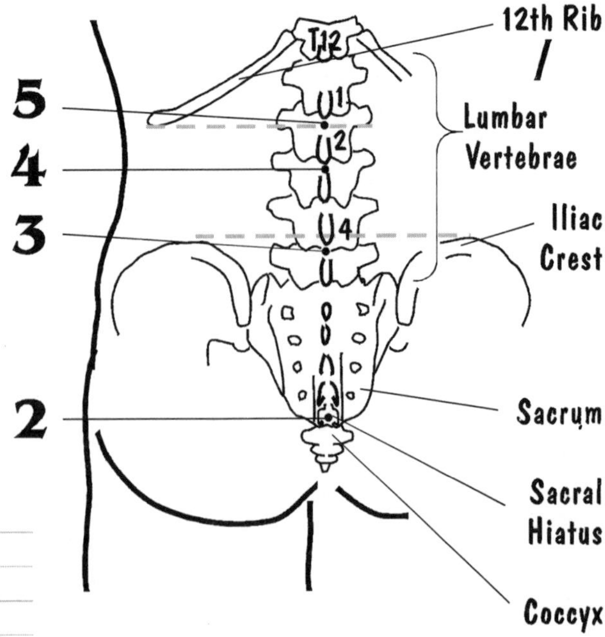

12th Rib

5

4

3

Lumbar
Vertebrae

Iliac
Crest

2

Sacrum

Sacral
Hiatus

Coccyx

Description:

~ Changqiang ~ GV(Du) 1

Location: Midway between the coccyx tip and the anus.
Basic Feature: 'Luo' connecting pt.. Interaction with K, CV(Ren) and some sources indicate also interaction with GB. Sea of marrow.
Note: ....

~ Yaoshu ~ GV(Du) 2

Location: In the center of the sacral hiatus.
Tips & References: Search for the sacral hiatus depression at the sacrum base, superior to the coccyx.
Note: ....

~ Yaoyangguan ~ GV(Du) 3

Location: Inferior to L4 spinous process.
Tips & References: Inferior to the iliac crest superior border line.
Note: ....

~ Mingmen ~ GV(Du) 4

Location: Inferior to L2 spinous process.
Note: ....

~ Xuanshu ~ GV(Du) 5

Location: Inferior to L1 spinous process.
Tips & References: Level with, or slightly inferior to the 12th rib free end.
Note: ....

Governing Vessel

notes:

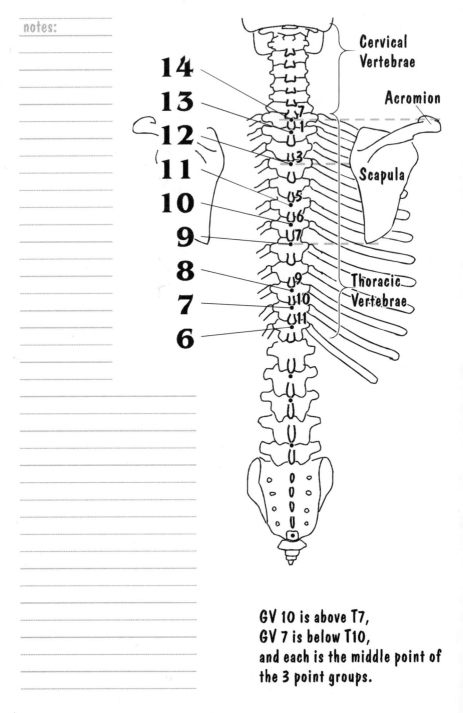

14
13
12
11
10
9
8
7
6

Cervical
Vertebrae

Acromion

Scapula

Thoracic
Vertebrae

GV 10 is above T7,
GV 7 is below T10,
and each is the middle point of
the 3 point groups.

Description:

~ Jizhong ~ GV(Du) 6

Location: Inferior to T11 spinous process.
Note: ....

~ Zhongshu ~ GV(Du) 7

Location: Inferior to T10 spinous process.
Note: ....

~ Jinsuo ~ GV(Du) 8

Location: Inferior to T9 spinous process.
Note: ....

~ Zhiyang ~ GV(Du) 9

Location: Inferior to T7 spinous process.
Tips & References: Level with the scapula's inferior edge.
Note: ....

~ Lingtai ~ GV(Du) 10

Location: Inferior to T6 spinous process.
Note: ....

~ Shendao ~ GV(Du) 11

Location: Inferior to T5 spinous process.
Note: ....

~ Shenzhu ~ GV(Du) 12

Location: Inferior to T3 spinous process.
☆ Level with the scapular spine medial end.
Note: ....

~ Taodao ~ GV(Du) 13

Location: Inferior to T1 spinous process.
Tips & References: T1 spinous process is the most extended process on the neck base. Search for the second process that can be felt when moving inferiorly along the neck midline (when the head is anteriorly dropped, T1 is the first spinous process to be felt).
Basic Feature: Interaction with UB.
Note: ....

~ Dazhui ~ GV(Du) 14

Location: Inferior to C7 spinous process.
Tips & References: Level with the acromion.
☆ Search for the first spinous process that can be felt when moving inferiorly along the neck midline (when the head is anteriorly dropped, it disappears).
Basic Feature: Interaction with six Yang meridians (LI, St, SI, UB, TW(SJ), GB).
Note: ....

Governing Vessel

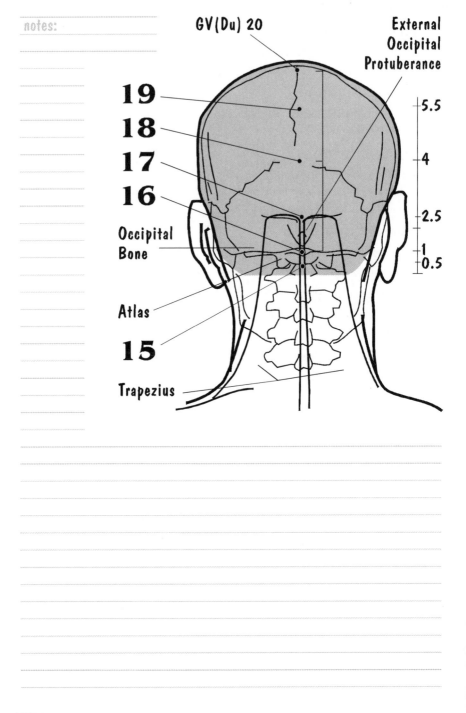

notes:

GV(Du) 20

External
Occipital
Protuberance

19

18

17

16

Occipital
Bone

5.5

4

2.5

1
0.5

Atlas

15

Trapezius

Description:

~ Yamen ~ GV(Du) 15

Location: 0.5 cun inferior to the external occipital protuberance.

Tips & References: Inferior to C1 (Atlas) spinous process.

☆ The atlas spinous process is hard to locate for it is deep and covered by complicated structure.

☆ 0.5 cun superior to the neck hairline* midpoint.

☆ 0.5 cun inferior to GV(Du) 16.

Basic Feature: Sea of Qi. Interaction with Yangwei (Ya-L).

Note: ....

~ Fengfu ~ GV(Du) 16

Location: Inferior to the external occipital protuberance (and the occipital bone).

Tips & References: Between the two trapezius muscles (of each side).

☆ 1 cun superior to the neck hairline* midpoint.

Basic Feature: Window to the Sky. Interaction with Yangwei (Ya-L) and some sources indicate also interaction with UB.

Note: ....

~ Naohu ~ GV(Du) 17

Location: Superior to the external occipital protuberance.

Tips & References: 2.5 cun superior to the neck hairline* midpoint.

☆ 1.5 cun superior to GV(Du) 16.

☆ 1/4 of the distance between GV(Du) 16 to GV(Du) 20.

Basic Feature: Many sources indicate interaction with UB.

Note: ....

~ Qiangjian ~ GV(Du) 18

Location: 4 cun superior to the neck hairline* midpoint.

Tips & References: 1.5 cun superior to GV(Du) 17.

☆ 3 cun posterior to GV(Du) 20.

☆ Midway between GV(Du) 16 to GV(Du) 20.

Note: ....

~ Houding ~ GV(Du) 19

Location: 5.5 cun superior to the neck hairline* midpoint.

☆ 3 cun superior to the external occipital protuberance

☆ 1.5 cun superior to GV(Du) 18.

☆ 3/4 of the distance between GV(Du) 16 to GV(Du) 20.

Note: ....

* The hairline is the borderline between a regular skin tissue and the oilier hair-skin tissue. This borderline can be felt when running the fingernail on the skin.

~ Points on Du Mai ~
Governing Vessel

notes:

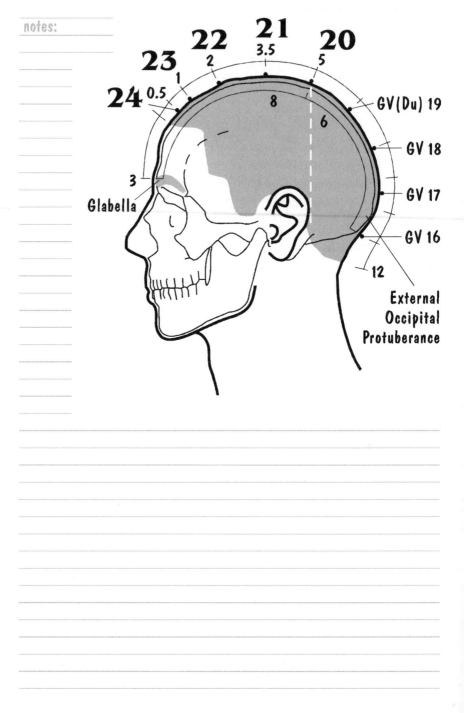

23 **22** **21** **20**
          2   3.5   5

24 0.5
        1

                              8   GV(Du) 19

                              6   GV 18

3   GV 17

Glabella

                                          GV 16

                                    12

                                    External
                                    Occipital
                                    Protuberance

Description:

~ Baihui ~ GV(Du) 20

Location: 7 cun superior to the neck hairline* midpoint.
Tips & References: 5 cun posterior to the forehead hairline midpoint.
☆ Midway, on the straight line that connects the two ear auricles' (helix) posterior borders.
☆ 8 cun posterior to the glabella and 6 cun superior to the external occipital protuberance inferior border.
☆ When reaching the point, in a posterior movement, it feels like stepping down from a flat surface.
Basic Feature: Sea of marrow. Many sources indicate interaction with UB and some indicate also interaction with all other Yang meridians and Liv.
Note: ....

~ Qianding ~ GV(Du) 21

Location: 3.5 cun posterior to the forehead hairline* midpoint.
Tips & References: 1.5 cun anterior to GV(Du) 20
Note: ....

~ Xinhui ~ GV(Du) 22

Location: 2 cun posterior to the forehead hairline* midpoint.
Tips & References: 1.5 cun posterior to GV(Du) 24, 3 cun anterior to GV(Du) 20.
Note: ....

~ Shangxing ~ GV(Du) 23

Location: 1 cun posterior to the forehead hairline* midpoint.
Tips & References: 0.5 cun posterior to GV(Du) 24.
Note: ....

~ Shenting ~ GV(Du) 24

Location: 0.5 cun posterior to the forehead hairline* midpoint.
Basic Feature: Interaction with St and UB.
Note: ....

* The hairline is the borderline between a regular skin tissue and the oilier hair-skin tissue. This borderline can be felt when running the fingernail on the skin.

Governing Vessel

notes:

25
26
27

1/3

Philatrum Skin

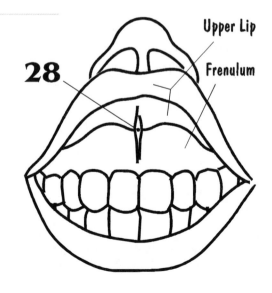

Upper Lip

Frenulum

28

Description:

~ Suliao ~ GV(Du) 25

Location: At the nose tip.
Note: ....

~ Shuigou ~ GV(Du) 26

Location: On the face midline, 1/3 of the distance between the nose root inferior border and the upper lip superior border.
Basic Feature: Interaction with LI and St.
Note: ....

~ Duiduan ~ GV(Du) 27

Location: Midpoint of the borderline between the upper lip and the philatrum skin.
Note: ....

~ Yinjiao ~ GV(Du) 28

Location: In the mouth, at the meeting of the upper gum (frenulum) with the upper lip.
Basic Feature: Interaction point with CV(Ren) and some sources indicate also interaction with St.
Note: ....

Points on
~ Chong Mai ~
Penetrating Vessel

Main Points:
☆ Starting: CV(Ren) 1
☆ Opening: Sp 4
☆ Coupled: P 6
☆ 'Xi' Accumulation: None
Abbreviation used in this guide: Pen.

Points on
~ Yinwei Mai ~
Yin Linking Vessel

Main Points:
☆ Starting: K 9
☆ Opening: P 6
☆ Coupled: Sp 4
☆ 'Xi' Accumulation: K 9
Abbreviation used in this guide: Yi-L.

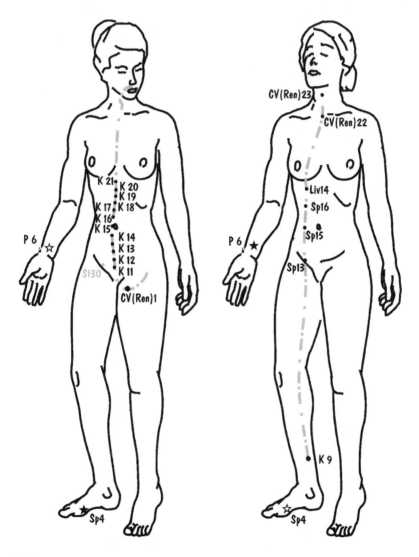

<table>
<tr><td>

Points on
~ Dai Mai ~
Girdle Vessel

</td><td>

Points on
~ Yangwei Mai ~
Yang Linking Vessel

</td></tr>
<tr><td>

Main Points:
☆ Starting: GB 26
☆ Opening: GB 41
☆ Coupled: TW(SJ) 5
☆ 'Xi' Accumulation: None
Abbreviation used in this guide: Gir.

</td><td>

Main Points:
☆ Starting: UB 63
☆ Opening: TW(SJ) 5
☆ Coupled: GB 41
☆ 'Xi' Accumulation: GB 35
Abbreviation used in this guide: Ya-L

</td></tr>
</table>

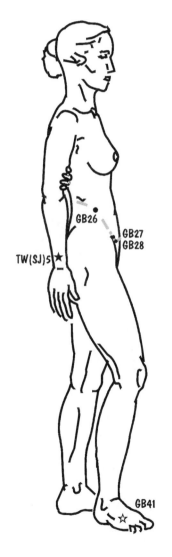

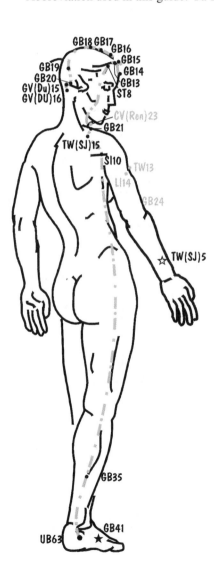

Points on
~ Yinqiao Mai ~
Yin Heel Vessel

Main Points:

☆ Starting: K 6
☆ Opening: K 6
☆ Coupled: Lu 7
☆ 'Xi' Accumulation: K 8

Abbreviation used in this guide: Yi-H

Points on
~ Yangqiao Mai ~
Yang Heel Vessel

Main Points:

☆ Starting: UB 62
☆ Opening: UB 62
☆ Coupled: SI 3
☆ 'Xi' Accumulation: UB 59

Abbreviation used in this guide: Ya-H

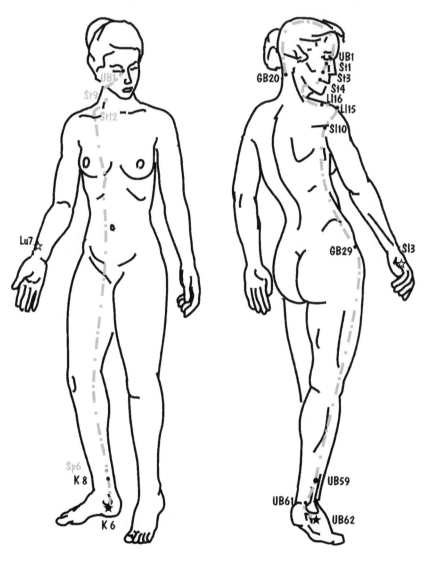

Points by Feature

~ Extra Meridians Main Points ~

	Chong Mai (Pen.)	Yinwei Mai (Yi-L)	Dai Mai (Gir.)	Yangwei Mai (Ya-L)
Starting	CV(Ren) 1	K 9	GB 26	UB 63
Opening	Sp 4	P 6	GB 41	TW(SJ) 5
Coupled	P 6	Sp 4	TW(SJ) 5	GB 41
'Xi' accumulation	---	K 9	---	GB 35

	Ren Mai (CV)	Yinqiao Mai (Yi-H)	Du Mai (GV)	Yangqiao Mai (Ya-H)
Starting	CV(Ren) 1	K 6	GV(Du) 1	UB 62
Opening	Lu 7	K 6	SI 3	UB 62
Coupled	K 6	Lu 7	UB 62	SI 3
'Xi' accumulation	---	K 8	---	UB 59
'Luo' Connecting	CV(Ren) 15	---	GV(Du) 1	---
Back 'Shu' Transporting	---	---	UB 16	---

~ Interaction Points with the Meridians ~

Lung (Lu): P5*.

Large Intestine (LI): St4, 12*, 37, SI12, TW(SJ)8*, 13*, GB4*, 5, 6, 14*, 21*, CV(Ren)24*, GV(Du)14, 20*, 26.

Stomach (St): LI20, Sp1, UB1, GB3, 4, 5*, 6, 14*, 39, CV(Ren)3*, 4*, 12, 24, 13, GV(Du) 14, 20*, 24, 26, 28*.

Spleen (Sp): Lu1, GB24, Liv14, CV(Ren)3, 4, 10, 17*.

Heart (H): P5*.

Small Intestine (SI): LI 14, 15*, St 12*, 39, UB 1, 11, 41, TW(SJ) 8*, 20*, 22, GB1, 11*, CV(Ren)17, 12, 13, GV(Du) 14, 20*.

Urinary Bladder (UB): LI14, St12*, SI10, GB7-11, 12,15, 23*, 30, 39, CV(Ren)17*, GV(Du)13, 14, 24, 16*, 17, 20.

Kidney (K): Sp6, UB58, CV(Ren)3, 4, 7, 17*, GV(Du)1.

Triple Warmer (TW/SJ): St12*, SI12, 18, 19, P1*, UB1*, 11, 39, GB1, 3, 4, 5*,6, 21, 11*, 14*, 20*,21, CV(Ren)12, 17*, GV(Du)14, 20*.

Gall Bladder (GB): LI15*, St7, 8, 9*, 12*, SI19, 12, P1, TW(SJ)15, 17, 20, 22, UB1*, 11, 33*, Liv1, 13, GV(Du)1, 14, 20*.

Liver (Liv): Sp6, 12, 13, P1, UB33*, CV(Ren)2-4, GV(Du)20*.

Conception Vessel (CV/Ren): St1, 4, GV(Du)1, 28*.

Governing Vessel (GV/Du): UB1*, 11*, 12, CV(Ren)1, 24*.

* These points are not indicated in some major sources.

~ Twelve Meridians Main Points ~

Yin Meridians	Lu	Sp	H	K	P	Liv
'Jing' Well / Wood	11	1	9 ⇑	1 ⇓	9 ⇑	1 ⊗
'Ying' Spring / Fire	10	2 ⇑	8 ⊗	2	8 ⊗	2 ⇓
'Shu' Stream / Earth	9 ⇑	3 ⊗	7 ⇓	3	7 ⇓	3
'Yuan' Source	**9**	**3**	**7**	**3**	**7**	**3**
'Jing' River / Metal	8 ⊗	5 ⇓	4	7 ⇑	5	4
'He' Sea / Water	5 ⇓	9	3	10 ⊗	3	8 ⇑
'Luo' Connecting	7	4	5	4	6	5
'Xi' Accumulation	6	8	6	5	4	6
Back 'Shu' Transporting	UB 13	UB 20	UB 15	UB 23	UB 14	UB 18
Front 'Mu' Collecting	Lu 1	Liv 13	CV 14	GB 25	CV 17	Liv 14
Dominant Hours	3-5 AM	9-11 AM	11AM-1P	5-7 PM	7-9 PM	1-3 AM

Yang Meridians	LI	St	SI	UB	TW-SJ	GB
'Jing' Well / Metal	1 ⊗	45 ⇓	1	67 ⇑	1	44
'Ying' Spring / Water	2 ⇓	44	2	66 ⊗	2	43 ⇑
'Shu' Stream / Wood	3	43	3 ⇑	65 ⇓	3 ⇑	41 ⊗
'Yuan' Source	**4**	**42**	**4**	**64**	**4**	**40**
'Jing' River / Fire	5	41 ⇑	5 ⊗	60	6 ⊗	38 ⇓
'He' Sea / Earth	11 ⇑	36 ⊗	8 ⇓	40	10 ⇓	34
'Luo' Connecting	6	40	7	58	5	37
'Xi' Accumulation	7	34	6	63	7	36
Back 'Shu' Transporting	UB 25	UB 21	UB 27	UB 28	UB 22	UB 19
Front 'Mu' Collecting	St 25	CV 12	CV 4	CV 3	CV 5	GB 24
Lower 'He' Sea	St 37	---	St 39	---	UB 39	---
Dominant Hours	5-7 AM	7-9 AM	1-3 PM	3-5 PM	9-11 PM	11PM-1A

⇑ for tonification (mother) point, ⇓ for sedation (son) point and ⊗ for horary point.

~ 'Hui' Gathering Points ~

Lu 9	UB 11	UB 17	GB 34	GB 39	Liv 13	CV12	CV17
Blood Vessels	Bones	Blood	Tendons	Bone Marrow	Zang~Yin Organs	Fu~Yang Organs	Qi

~ Command Points ~

Lu 7	LI 4	St 36	UB 40
Head & Nape	Face & Mouth	Abdomen	Lumbar & Back

~ Points of Four Seas ~

Sea of Qi	St 9 : ....
	UB 10 : ....
	CV(Ren) 17 : ....
	GV(Du) 15 : ....
Sea of Blood	St 37 : ....
	St 39 : ....
	UB 11 : ....
	CV(Ren) 4 : ....
Sea of Nourishment	St 30 : ....
	St 36 : ....
Sea of Marrow	GV(Du) 16 : ....
	GV(Du) 20 : ....

~ Points of Window to the Sky ~

Lu 3 : ....

LI 18 : ....

St 9 : ....

SI 16 : ....

SI 17 : ....

UB 10 : ....

P 1 : ....

TW(SJ) 16 : ....

CV(Ren) 22: ....

GV(Du) 16 / 15 : ....

Source List for Alternative Point Locations

Most of the points are similarly located throughout the various written sources, but some points are located differently in one or a few of them. The following is a list of points shown in this guide with alternative location and their sources.

UB 63, GB16-18, GB22-23: The Location of Acupoints / State Standard of the Peoples' Republic of China.

Sp 21, UB 62, GB 11: A Manual of Acupuncture / P. Deadman, M. Al-Khafaji, Kevin B..

K 11-21: 'Zhen Jiu Da Cheng': The Great Comparison of Acupuncture and Moxibustion.

LI 20, Sp 5, K 1, Liv 8: The Book of Acupuncture Points / James Tin Yau So.

SI 11, UB 4: 'Jia Yi': A-B classic of Acupuncture and Moxibustion.

P 9: 'Jin Jia': Gold Mirror of Orthodox Medical Lineage.

Map of Hand Points

~ Anterior-Palmar View ~ Lateral-Dorsal View ~

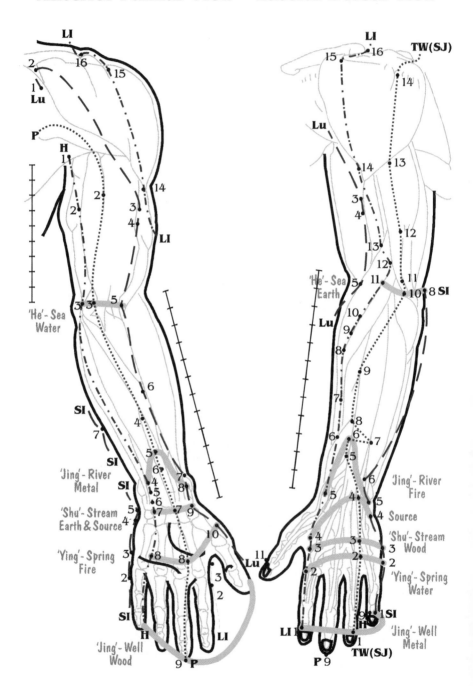

~ Posterior-Ulnar View ~

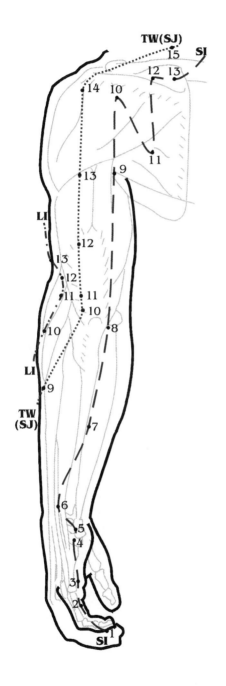

Map of Leg Points

~ Superior View ~ ~ Medial View ~

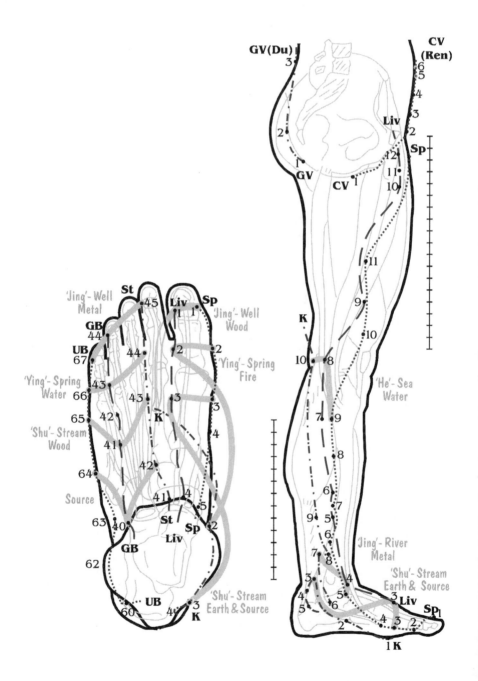

~ Acupoint Location Guide ~

~Anterior View ~Lateral View ~Posterior View~

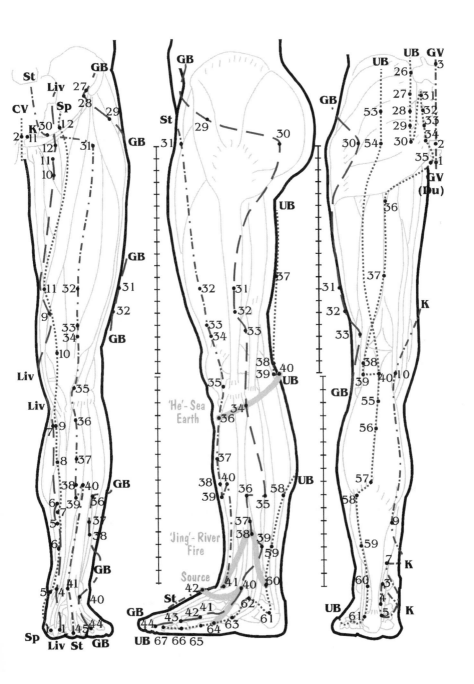

Map of Torso Points

~ Superior View ~   ~ Anterior View ~

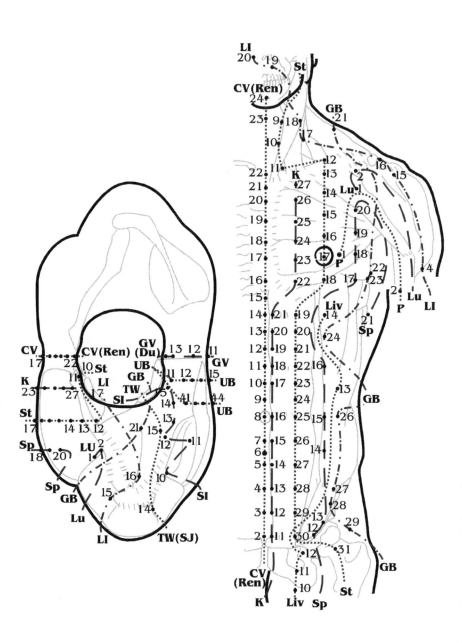

~ Acupoint Location Guide ~

~ Lateral View ~   ~ Posterior View ~

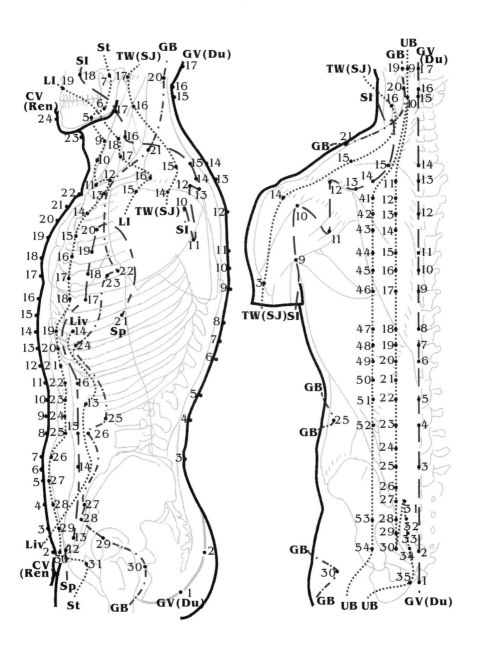

Map of Head Points

~ Different Views ~

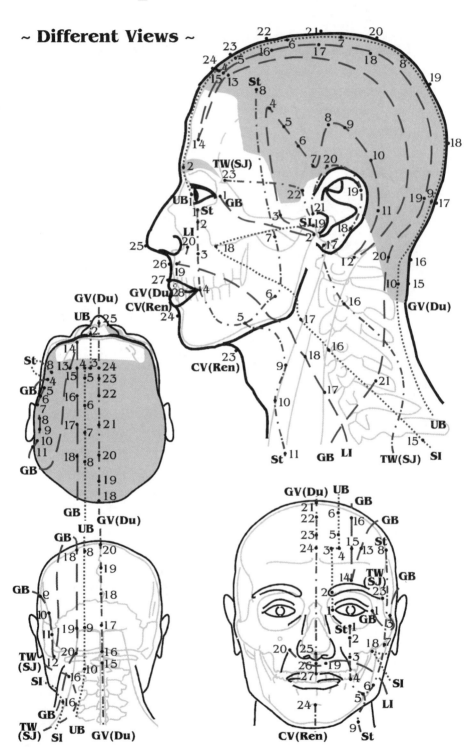

~ Acupoint Location Guide ~

Point Index

L...

Liangqiu ~ **St 34** (P. 44)
Lianquan ~ **CV(Ren) 23** (p. 162)
Lidui ~ **St 45** (p. 48)
Lieque ~ **Lu 7** (p. 18)
Ligou~ **Liv 5** (p. 152)
Lingdao ~ **H 4** (p. 62)
Lingtai ~ **GV(Du) 10** (p. 166)
Lingxu ~ **K 24** (p. 110)
Lougu ~ **Sp 7** (p. 52)
Luoque ~ **UB 8** (p. 78)
Luxi ~ **TW(SJ) 19** (p. 124)

~ M ~

Meichong ~ **UB 3** (p. 76)
Mingmen ~ **GV(Du) 4** (p. 164)
Muchuang ~ **GB 16** (p. 134)

~ N ~

Naohu ~ **GV(Du) 17** (p. 168)
Naohui ~ **TW(SJ) 13** (p. 120)
Naokong ~ **GB 19** (p. 136)
Naoshu ~ **SI 10** (p. 70)
Neiguan ~ **P 6** (p. 112)
Neiting ~ **St 44** (p. 48)

~ P ~

Pangguangshu ~ **UB 28** (p. 84)
Pianli ~ **LI 6** (p. 26)
Pishu ~ **UB 20** (p. 82)
Pohu ~ **UB 42** (p. 90)
Pucan ~ **UB 61** (p. 96)

~ Q ~

Qianding ~ **GV(Du) 21** (p. 170)
Qiangjian ~ **GV(Du) 18** (p. 168)
Qiangu ~ **SI 2** (p. 66)
Qichong ~ **St 30** (p. 42)

Q...

Qihai ~ **CV(Ren) 6** (p. 156)
Qihaishu ~ **UB 24** (p. 82)
Qihu ~ **St 13** (p. 38)
Qimai ~ **TW(SJ) 18** (p. 124)
Qimen ~ **Liv 14** (p. 154)
Qinglengyuan ~ **TW(SJ)11** (p.120)
Qingling ~ **H 2** (p. 60)
Qishe ~ **St 11** (p. 36)
Qiuxu ~ **GB 40** (p. 148)
Qixue ~ **K 13** (p. 106)
Quanliao ~ **SI 18** (p. 74)
Qubin ~ **GB 7** (p. 130)
Quchai ~ **UB 4** (p. 78)
Quchi ~ **LI 11** (p. 26)
Quepen ~ **St 12** (p. 38)
Qugu ~ **CV(Ren) 2** (p. 156)
Ququan ~ **Liv 8** (p. 152)
Quyuan ~ **SI 13** (p. 72)
Quze ~ **P 3** (p. 112)

~ R ~

Rangu ~ **K 2** (p. 100)
Renying ~ **St 9** (p. 36)
Renzhong ~ **GV(Du) 26** (p. 172)
Riyue ~ **GB 24** (p. 138)
Rugen ~ **St 18** (p. 38)
Ruzhong ~ **St 17** (p. 38)

~ S ~

Sanjian ~ **LI 3** (p. 22)
Sanjiaoshu ~ **UB 22** (p. 82)
Sanyangluo ~ **TW(SJ) 8** (p. 118)
Sanyinjiao ~ **Sp 6** (p. 52)
Shangguan ~ **GB 3** (p. 128)
Shangjuxu ~ **St 37** (p. 46)
ShangLian ~ **LI 9** (p. 26)
Shangliao ~ **UB 31** (p. 86)

S...

Shangqiu ~ Sp 5 (p. 52)

Shangqu ~ K 17 (p. 108)

Shangwan ~ CV(Ren) 13 (p. 158)

Shangxing ~ GV(Du) 23 (p. 170)

Shangyang ~ LI 1 (p. 22)

Shaochong ~ H 9 (p. 64)

Shaofu ~ H 8 (p. 64)

Shaohai ~ H 3 (p. 60)

Shaoshang ~ Lu 11 (p. 20)

Shaoze ~ SI 1 (p. 66)

Shencang ~ K 25 (p. 110)

Shendao ~ GV(Du) 11 (p. 166)

Shenfeng ~ K 23 (p. 110)

Shenmai ~ UB 62 (p. 96)

Shenmen ~ H 7 (p. 64)

Shenque ~ CV(Ren) 8 (p. 156)

Shenshu ~ UB 23 (p. 82)

Shentang ~ UB 44 (p. 90)

Shenting ~ GV(Du) 24 (p. 170)

Shenzhu ~ GV(Du) 12 (p. 166)

Shidou ~ Sp 17 (p. 58)

Shiguan ~ K 18 (p. 108)

Shimen ~ CV(Ren) 5 (p. 156)

Shousanli ~ LI 10 (p. 26)

Shouwuli ~ LI 13 (p. 28)

Shuaigu ~ GB 8 (p. 130)

Shufu ~ K 27 (p. 110)

Shugu ~ UB 65 (p. 98)

Shuidao ~ St 28 (p. 42)

Shuifen ~ CV(Ren) 9 (p. 158)

Shuigou ~ GV(Du) 26 (p. 172)

Shuiquan ~ K 5 (p. 102)

Shuitu ~ St 10 (p.36)

Sibai ~ St 2 (p. 32)

Sidu ~ TW(SJ) 9 (p. 118)

Siman ~ K 14 (p. 106)

Suliao ~ GV(Du) 25 (p. 172)

~ T ~

Taibai ~ Sp 3 (p. 50)

Taichong ~ Liv 3 (p. 150)

Taixi ~ K 3 (p. 102)

Taiyi ~ St 23 (p. 40)

Taiyuan ~ Lu 9 (p. 20)

Taodao ~ GV(Du) 13 (p. 166)

Tianchi ~ P 1 (p. 112)

Tianchong ~ GB 9 (p. 130)

Tianchuang ~ SI 16 (p. 72)

Tianding ~ LI 17 (p. 30)

Tianfu ~ Lu 3 (p. 16)

Tianjing ~ TW(SJ) 10 (p. 120)

Tianliao ~ TW(SJ) 15 (p. 122)

Tianquan ~ P 2 (p. 112)

Tianrong ~ SI 17 (p. 72)

Tianshu ~ St 25 (p. 42)

Tiantu ~ CV(Ren) 22 (p. 160)

Tianxi ~ Sp 18 (p. 58)

Tianyou ~ TW(SJ) 16 (p. 122)

Tianzhu ~ UB 10 (p. 78)

Tianzong ~ SI 11 (p. 70)

Tiaokou ~ St 38 (p. 46)

Tinggong ~ SI 19 (p. 74)

Tinghui ~ GB 2 (p. 128)

Tongli ~ H 5 (p. 62)

Tongtian ~ UB 7 (p. 78)

Tongziliao ~ GB 1 (p. 128)

Toulinqi ~ GB 15 (p. 134)

Touqiaoyin ~ GB 11 (p. 132)

Touwei ~ St 8 (p. 34)

~ W ~

Waiguan ~ TW(SJ) 5 (p. 118)

Wailing ~ St 26 (P. 42)

Waiqiu ~ GB 36 (p. 146)

Wangu ~ GB 12 (p. 132)

Wangu ~ SI 4 (p. 66)

W...

Weicang ~ UB 50 (p. 92)
Weidao ~ GB 28 (p. 140)
Weishu ~ UB 21 (p. 82)
Weiyang ~ UB 39 (p. 88)
Weizhong ~ UB 40 (p. 88)
Wenliu ~ LI 7 (p. 26)
Wuchu ~ UB 5 (p. 78)
Wushu ~ GB 27 (p. 140)
Wuyi ~ St 15 (p. 38)

~ X ~

Xiabai ~ Lu 4 (p. 16)
Xiaguan ~ St 7 (p. 34)
Xiajuxu ~ St 39 (p. 46)
Xialian ~ LI 8 (p. 26)
Xialiao ~ UB 34 (p. 86)
Xiangu ~ St 43 (p. 48)
Xiaochangshu ~ UB 27 (p. 84)
Xiaohai ~ SI 8 (p. 68)
Xiaoluo ~ TW(SJ) 12 (p. 120)
Xiawan ~ CV(Ren) 10 (p. 158)
Xiaxi ~ GB 43 (p. 148)
Xiguan ~ Liv 7 (p. 152)
Ximen ~ P 4 (p. 112)
Xingjian ~ Liv 2 (p. 150)
Xinhui ~ GV(Du) 22 (p. 170)
Xinshu ~ UB 15 (p. 80)
Xiongxiang ~ Sp 19 (p. 58)
Xiyangguan ~ GB 33 (p. 144)
Xuanji ~ CV(Ren) 21 (p. 160)
Xuanli ~ GB 6 (p. 130)
Xuanlu ~ GB 5 (p. 130)
Xuanshu ~ GV(Du) 5 (p. 164)
Xuanzhong ~ GB 39 (p. 146)
Xuehai ~ Sp 10 (p. 54)

~ Y ~

Yamen ~ GV(Du) 15 (p. 168)
Yangbai ~ GB 14 (p. 132)
Yangchi ~ TW(SJ) 4 (p. 118)
Yangfu ~ GB 38 (p. 146)
Yanggang ~ UB 48 (p. 92)
Yanggu ~ SI 5 (p. 66)
Yangjiao ~ GB 35 (p. 146)
Yanglao ~ SI 6 (p. 68)
Yanglingquan ~ GB 34 (p.146)
Yangxi ~ LI 5 (p. 24)
Yaoshu ~ GV(Du) 2 (p. 164)
Yaoyangguan ~GV(Du) 3 (p.164)
Yemen ~ TW(SJ) 2 (p. 116)
Yifeng ~ TW(SJ) 17 (p. 124)
Yinbai ~ Sp 1 (p.50)
Yinbao ~ Liv 9 (p. 154)
Yindu ~ K 19 (p. 108)
Yingchuang ~ St 16 (p. 38)
Yingu ~ K 10 (p. 104)
Yingxiang ~ LI 20 (p. 30)
Yinjiao ~ CV(Ren) 7 (p. 156)
Yinjiao ~ GV(Du) 28 (p. 172)
Yinlian ~ Liv 11 (p. 154)
Yinlingquan ~ Sp 9 (p. 52)
Yinmen ~ UB 37 (p. 88)
Yinshi ~ St 33 (p. 44)
Yinxi ~ H 6 (p. 62)
Yishe ~ UB 49 (p. 92)
Yixi ~ UB 45 (p. 90)
Yongquan ~ K 1 (p. 100)
Youmen ~ K 21 (p. 108)
Yuanye ~ GB 22 (p. 138)
Yuji ~ Lu 10 (p. 20)
Yunmen ~ Lu 2 (p. 16)
Yutang ~ CV(Ren) 18 (p. 160)
Yuzhen ~ UB 9 (p. 78)
Yuzhong ~ K 26 (p. 110)

~ Z ~

Zhongliao ~ UB 33 (p. 86)

Zhonglushu ~ UB 29 (p. 84)

Zhongshu ~ GV(Du) 7 (p. 166)

Zhongting ~ CV(Ren) 16 (p. 160)

Zhongwan ~ CV(Ren) 12 (p. 158)

Zhongzhu ~ TW(SJ) 3 (p. 116)

Zhongzhu ~ K 15 (p. 106)

Zhourong ~ Sp 20 (p. 58)

Zhouliao ~ LI 12 (p. 28)

Zhubin ~ K 9 (p. 104)

Zanzhu ~ UB 2 (p. 76)

Zigong ~ CV(Ren) 19 (p. 160)

Zulinqi ~ GB 41 (p. 148)

Zuqiaoyin ~ GB 44 (p. 148)

Zusanli ~ St 36 (p. 46)

Zutonggu ~ UB 66 (p. 98)

Zuwuli ~ Liv 10 (p. 154)

Zhangmen ~ Liv 13 (p. 154)

Zhaohai ~ K 6 (p. 102)

Zhejin ~ GB 23 (p. 138)

Zhengying ~ GB 17 (p. 134)

Zhigou ~ TW(SJ) 6 (p. 118)

Zhizheng ~ SI 7 (p. 68)

Zhibian ~ UB 54 (p. 94)

Zhishi ~ UB 52 (p. 92)

Zhiyang ~ GV(Du) 9 (p. 166)

Zhiyin ~ UB 67 (p. 98)

Zhongchong ~ P 9 (p. 114)

Zhongdu ~ Liv 6 (p. 152)

Zhongdu ~ GB 32 (p. 144)

Zhongfeng ~ Liv 4 (p. 150)

Zhongfu ~ Lu 1 (p. 16)

Bibliography

Essentials of Chinese Acupuncture / Foreign Languages Press, Beijing / 1993.

Chinese Acupuncture and Moxibustion / Cheng Xinnong / Foreign Languages Press, Beijing / 1996.

The Location of Acupoints / State Standard of the Peoples' Republic of China / Foreign Languages Press, Beijing / 1990.

The Book of Acupuncture Points / James Tin Yau So / Paradigm Publication / 1984.

A Manual of Acupuncture / Peter Deadman, Mazin Al-Khafaji, Kevin Baker / Journal of Chinese Medicine Publication / 1998.

The Foundations of Chinese Medicine / Giovanni Maciocia / Churchill Livingstone / 1989.

Anatomical Topography / Ofer Raz / 1995.

Grasping the Wind / Andrew Ellis, Nigel Wiseman, Ken Boss / Paradigm Publication / 1989.

Acupuncture / Felix Mann / Vintage Books / 1972.

Color Atlas of Anatomy / Johannes W. Rohen, Chihiro Yokochi / IGAKU-SHOIN / 1993.

The Anatomy Coloring Book / Wynn Kapit, Lawrence M. Elson / Harper Collins Publishers / 1977.